THE COMP

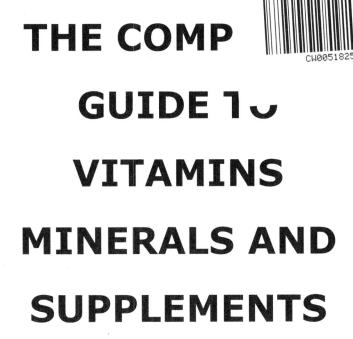
CW00518259

GUIDE TO

VITAMINS

MINERALS AND

SUPPLEMENTS

The New 2020 Essential
A To Z Guide Book

Robin A. Miller

Table of Contents

DISCLAIMER 5

© COPYRIGHT 2019 MELWEB MARKETING 5

INTRODUCTION 6

VITAMIN ORIGINS 8

VITAMIN C 13

VITAMIN E 33

LIPOIC ACID 38

    B Vitamins *40*

VITAMIN B1 40

VITAMIN B2 43

VITAMIN B3 (NIACIN) 45

VITAMIN B6 56

VITAMIN B7 (BIOTIN) 59

VITAMIN B9 (FOLIC ACID) 62

    Fat Soluble Vitamins *67*

VITAMIN A 67

VITAMIN K 71

VITAMIN D 73

    Other Vitamins *80*

CHOLINE 80

INOSITOL 82

PABA (PARA- AMINO BENZOIC ACID) 83

AMINO ACIDS 84

    Essential Amino Acids *85*

HISTIDINE 85

ISOLEUCINE 86

VALINE 86

LYSINE 87

METHIONINE 88

PHENYLALANINE 89

THREONINE 90

TRYPTOPHAN 91

Non-Essential Amino Acids *92*

ALANINE 92

ARGININE 93

ASPARTIC ACID 95

CARNITINE 95

CARNOSINE 96

CYSTEINE 97

GLUTAMIC ACID 98

GLYCINE 100

ORNITHINE 101

PROLINE 102

SERINE 103

TAURINE 104

TYROSINE 105

Minerals *106*

BORON 106

CALCIUM 107

CHROMIUM 109

COPPER 110

IRON 112

MAGNESIUM 113

MANGANESE 121

3

MOLYBDENUM 123

POTASSIUM 124

SELENIUM 127

ZINC 129

Honorable Mentions Supplements 133

COQ10 133

CURCUMIN 137

FISH OIL 140

SKIN 141

RESVERATROL 144

Control Group Had A Healthy Diet 145

CONCLUSION 147

BELOW ARE A FEW OF OUR HIGHLY RECOMMENDED WEIGHT LOSS PRODUCTS WHICH ARE WORTH CHECKING OUT. 151

Disclaimer

The information contained in this guide is for informational purposes only. The author has made every effort to ensure the validity of the information provided in this Book, but it is NOT intended as medical advice and should not be used as a substitute for professional medical advice or treatment.

Introduction

Your body is composed of approximately 50 trillion cells depending on your body type and size. These cells are specific to the organ function. From epithelial or skin cells (which regulate body temperature and keep infection out) to hundreds of thousands of muscle cells), (skeletal, cardiac and smooth). From the 100 billion neurons in the mere three pound human brain, to the 100,000+ miles of blood vessels (enough to circle the world almost 5 times)!

This vast nervous system transmits information electrically and chemically at incredible speeds (up to 350 feet per second) to the rest of the body. From gametes, sex cells--- the sperm and egg----- to the creation of life itself.

This complex mechanism of our body and its panoply of cells works together to keep this intricate and complex machine running smoothly.

All cells die, however as they die, they are also being replaced. Vitamins, minerals and amino acids help with the repair and creation of these cells. The cells are composed of atoms and they are further broken down to a nucleus and electron. When an electron escapes, it is called a free radical. This is what happens when our body breaks down food to give us energy. The result is the oxidation of our DNA. This is essentially the basic theory behind the free radical theory of aging. A good example is a partially eaten apple. You will see that the apple quickly turns brown--- this browning or rotting is oxidation. To fight this oxidation, we need free radical scavengers, of which vitamins play a critical role. They work together in order to restore the cells balance and help the integration and communication among the cells as well as to help in replacing old cells with new cells.

The average male loses 96 million cells per minute and at the same time, as 96 million cells are dying; 96 million cells are being created.

For example, white blood cells last thirteen days, skin cells; thirty days, red blood cells; one hundred twenty days and liver cells are lost and replaced every eighteen months. The idea behind this book is to supplement your body with all the raw materials it needs to rebuild these cells as well as nutrients that can help you avoid serious health issues.

As they say, "you can't fight mother nature". You can't starve the body of vital organic nutrients it needs for replicating cells and rebuilding this complex machine without there being some eventual consequences.

Vitamin Origins

Supplementation has been the premise I have lived by and I know it has helped. I am in an advanced age group (60's) and I take no prescription medications at all.

Although there is no definitive answer it is more of my story which I think will help you to live as long as possible, as healthy as possible, and to achieve a quality of life that you truly deserve.

In subsequent chapters, we will delve into the specifics of supplementation, the benefits and the pitfalls.

My belief is that the benefits outweigh the negatives 10 to 1. I would rather spend a small amount now, rather than a giant amount later. An ounce of prevention in this case is worth more than one hundred pounds of cure.

Over 100 years ago, British Biochemist, Dr. Fredrick Hopkins showed the correlation between what he called "accessory food factors" and the human body. The body does not only need what are now known as macro-nutrients - protein, carbohydrates, minerals, water and fats but also needs micro-nutrients- "accessory factors". These later turned out to be vitamins. Most vitamins come from the diet or other sources as the body cannot synthesize them, two exceptions being vitamin D and biotin.

The skin can make Vitamin D when it is exposed to sunlight. However, people staying indoors and using sunscreen keep the vitamin from being produced and consequently some individuals may become deficient in vitamin D.

Biotin is created in the intestine from (friendly bacteria) but the exact amounts created are difficult to measure.

The word vitamin was coined in 1912 by Polish born American biochemist Casimir Funk who was investigating beriberi, a disease that causes depression, fatigue and nerve damage. He discovered an organic compound in rice husks that treated the illness. This compound was called B1 or thiamine. He called his discovery vitamine from the Latin word for "life" (vita) and amine because it was thought that these substances were amines (derivatives of ammonia). It was later discovered they were not so, therefore, the name was modified and the word "vitamin" was adopted.

Further vitamin research lead to many more vitamins being found. Vitamin K was discovered in 1929, vitamin C in 1932 and vitamin B12, 1948.

Casimir Funk later developed a theory along with Sir Frederick Hopkins called the "the vitamin hypothesis of deficiency" which explained how certain diseases such as scurvy or rickets can be prevented with proper vitamin consumption. Vitamins are essential for our health but we also need minerals such as iron, magnesium and calcium to remain healthy. All of these nutrients work synergistically with each other such as vitamin C and vitamin E.

Our primitive ancestors had great instincts in eating liver and intestines of the animals they killed. These micro-nutrients present in the specific body parts kept them fairly healthy. Today, thanks to modern science, we no longer have to resort to these barbaric practices.

There are two major categories of common vitamins: fat soluble and water soluble.

There are 4 Fat soluble vitamins are A, D, E and K. The water-soluble vitamins are B and C. There are eight vitamins in the B complex category: Riboflavin (B1), Thiamine (B2), Niacin (B3), Pantothenic acid (B5), Pyridoxine (B6), B12, Biotin and Folic acid.

One sulfur derived antioxidant is alpha lipoic acid. This supplement is unique because it is both fat and water soluble and readily crosses the blood brain barrier, increasing its availability to the body.

Water soluble vitamins easily dissolve in water and they will be excreted in the urine roughly 3 – 4 hours after ingestion. Therefore, I recommend that you ingest your water-soluble vitamin doses 3 to 4 times daily so that you can have a consistent serum level of these important vitamins.

Vitamin C

The big daddy of the water-soluble vitamins is vitamin C. The actual discovery of vitamin C is attributed to the Hungarian American Physiologist Albert Szent-Gyorgyi who in 1937 was awarded a noble laureate for the discovery of vitamin C and the citric acid cycle.

According to the Linus Pauling Institute: "Vitamin C is the primary water-soluble, non-enzymatic antioxidant in plasma and tissues. Even in small amounts vitamin C can protect indispensable molecules in the body, such as proteins, lipids (fats), carbohydrates, and nucleic acids (DNA and RNA), from damage by free radicals and reactive oxygen species (ROS) that are generated during normal metabolism, by active immune cells, and through exposure to toxins and pollutants..."

Scurvy killed many people before it was discovered in 1747 by Scottish Dr. James Lind that eating citrus prevented this disease. You should know that it was the vitamin C in the citrus that saved the day.

The importance of vitamin C is further shown by the fact that during pregnancy, the developing fetus will take vitamin C from the mother to further its development. Also, in one other study I came across regarding preterm rupture of membranes which can cause miscarriage, vitamin C supplementation, in such cases resulted in far fewer incidents in women who had a history of this dangerous condition.

Vitamin C is excellent for cell repair, circulation, wound healing and it also helps combat some of the negative effects of smoking and oral contraceptive use. So if you are a smoker it is critical to take adequate doses of this vitamin.

Bone forming cells called osteoblasts are stimulated to develop from precursor cells with vitamin C. Therefore, vitamin C will help with bone health. Osteoclasts which breakdown bone are actually inhibited by vitamin C. The health of the bone and the re-building of bone is improved with this vitamin and conversely, a deficiency accelerates bone loss.

Vitamin C forms a protein that makes collagen (the connective tissue between cells), skin, tendons, ligaments and blood vessels. More is needed during times of stress as stress can diminish the effectiveness of this vital micro-nutrient. Interestingly, animals who synthesize this vitamin can make up to 13 times the normal amount during stressful episodes.

Vitamin C helps to dilate blood vessels and also strengthens them. It helps to reduce the risk of cataracts and in general will help to protect vision. A recent study showed that women who took the supplement for 10 years were 23% less likely to develop cataracts, whereas 60% of the cataracts were seen in women who had not been taking the supplement.

Studies have also shown that there is less likelihood of cardiovascular events, (i.e. stroke, heart attack) with higher than RDA recommended doses. A ten year study by epidemiologist Dr. James Enstrom with men who took 300 mg or more per day of vitamin C had less heart disease and lived 6 years longer than the control group which took only 50 mg per day or less. In another study, 11,200 elderly were given hi-potency C which helped to reduce their mortality by 42%.

This study speaks to the fact that our arteries are lined with fibers made of the protein collagen, strengthening these walls and preventing tears in the arterial lining helps to prevent blockages. Vitamin C aids in wound healing and would also be a benefit post-operatively.

I'm sure when you had your last physical; your Doctor checked your cholesterol levels. HDL is the good cholesterol and LDL is the bad cholesterol. A good total cholesterol level including HDL and LDL should be below 200 mg/dl defined as milligrams per 10th of a liter. A liter is approximately 33.8 ounces.

According to the US natural library of medicine article regarding thirteen randomized controlled trials published between 1970 and June 2007. From the 13 trials, 14 separate group populations with hyper-cholesterolemia (high cholesterol) who were supplemented with at least 500 mg/dl of vitamin C for between 3 and 24 weeks were entered into the meta-analysis. This meta-analysis used a random-effects model; and the overall effect sizes were calculated for changes in LDL and HDL cholesterol, and triglyceride concentrations. The end result: supplementing with a minimum of 500 mg of vitamin C for at the minimum of 4 weeks resulted in a decrease in serum LDL cholesterol and triglycerides enough to reduce coronary heart risk by 11%. This is one more study which shows just how important taking this vitamin is.

We homo-sapiens along with other primates and guinea pigs don't make vitamin C. There is a theory that there is a defect in our genetic makeup that won't allow us to make vitamin C. For whatever reason, humans don't make vitamin C. A typical 155 pound billy goat makes roughly 13 grams of vitamin C a day- that is 13000 mg! The very famous Dr. Linus Pauling took 10 grams per day, eventually did get cancer but lived to be 93 years old! Thus, outliving many of his major critics some of whom died in their 60's.

In the very well-respected journal called Nature. Chinese Doctors did a meta-analysis of over 8,000 lung cancer survivors and concluded that for every 100 mg increase in vitamin C intake the incidence of lung cancer was 7% less. They concluded that a higher intake of vitamin C was related to a lesser risk of contracting lung cancer.

This powerful vitamin is good for vision, (nerve cells in the eyes require vitamin C in order to function properly, according to the journal of neuroscience from Oregon Health and Science University). Researchers used goldfish retina's which are similar in structure to the human eye, and showed that ascorbic acid could be neuro protective for the retina. Henrique Gersdoff, PH.D senior scientist and co-author of the study found that cells in the retina need to be bathed in high doses of C inside and out to function properly. Further researchers found that when the body is deprived of this vitamin, the concentration stays in the brain longer than anywhere else.

GABA receptors which act like a braking system on excitatory neurons stopped functioning when they were deprived of vitamin C which really shows how important this vitamin is and why the RDA of 60 mg is inadequate. Vitamin C may help preserve the receptor cells from premature breakdown. These findings could help glaucoma and epilepsy as both are caused by dysfunction of nerve cells in the retina and brain that become over excited due to the GABA receptors breaking down and not functioning in response to the lack of this vitamin.

(Allosteric modulation of retinal GABA receptors by ascorbic acid journal of neuroscience 2011).

Interestingly one of the symptoms of scurvy is depression which could be caused by lack of vitamin C. This amazing vitamin strengthens the immune system, can lower bad cholesterol and helps with blood vessel integrity as it fortifies the collagen or connective tissue.

Researches in Sweden discovered that vitamin C can dissolve toxic protein aggregates that build up in Alzheimer's' patients. (Caballero, E. Vickers, G.Moraga).

Further, vitamin C reduces tumor weight and growth rate by 50% in mouse models of brain, ovarian, and pancreatic cancers. The vitamin forms hydrogen peroxide in the extra cellular fluid surrounding the cancerous tumors. Hydrogen peroxide helps to kill the cancer cells as cancer cells ae not able to neutralize the hydrogen peroxide. Normal cells were not affected. (Science daily 5 august 2008).

Sepsis is a bacterial infection which has a high mortality rate in infants and the elderly. In this condition small blood clots form, blocking blood flow to vital organs, plugging the capillaries.

Vitamin C prevents this capillary plugging for up to 24 hours after injection (bio-factors 2009). They think this is accomplished by the ability of ascorbic acid to stimulate endothelial proliferation and further protecting nitric oxide which has a beneficial effect on the endothelium. (These line the cavities of the heart, blood and lymph vessels. This has lead researchers to the recommendation of ascorbic acid given intravenously to sepsis patients as an additional form of therapy.

Extra C may also help control the common cold, chicken pox, hepatitis, influenza, viral pneumonia, measles, mumps, polio and tuberculosis.

As far as polio is concerned, a debt of gratitude is owed to the great bacteriologist, Dr. Claus Jungeblut. Dr. Jungeblut, in 1935, published that ascorbic acid was prevention and cure for poliomyelitis and also inactivated the diphtheria and tetanus toxin.

As a biologist and statistician, Dr. Jungeblut discovered that those with polio had low levels of this vitamin, which in turn lead him to a mega dose treatment of polio using vitamin C. Unfortunately, those doctors tried to duplicate the results but were not successful. Some scientists say the reason is that they did not use a high enough dose of this vitamin.

One doctor who did believe in the validity of Dr. Jungebluts research, was Dr. Klenner. In 1949 Dr. Klenner found vitamin C to be effective in cold sores, fever blisters, shingles and viral meningitis.

Vitamin C also helps to detoxify hydrocarbons, nitrosamines and other cancer-causing chemicals. Vitamin C does not seem to work in chronic conditions such as aids but will augment the effects of more traditional ant-microbial agents.

Dr. Linus Pauling (twice a noble laureate winner) believed strongly that vitamin C can prevent or even slow the development of cancer. Cancer cells can hide from the body's own defensive mechanisms by forming a literal cocoon. Interestingly of the animals that do make their own vitamin C such as that billy goat we mentioned earlier, create this vitamin in the liver from glucose. Cancer exists on glucose and vitamin C is close enough to glucose (chemically) to fool the cancer into thinking it is receiving this nourishment when it is actually bringing the Trojan horse of vitamin C into its cells which may help the body to identify, slow and even kill these malicious cells.

The way it does this is by neutralizing hydrogen peroxide and turning it into H_2O_2, a harmless water vapor. Cancers do not contain catalase which would break down hydrogen peroxide so vitamin C helps to rid the normal cells of this oxidative chemical.

Many cancer patients die eventually from pneumonia, in a study by Pitt and Costrini (1979) half of a group of 800 marine recruits in a training camp were given 2 grams of vitamin C per day versus a placebo during an 8 week period, the result was that the placebo group, (not given vitamin C) were 7 times more likely to develop pneumonia than the group given the vitamin C supplement.

One of the many problems of cancer proliferation is that the cancer hides from the watch dogs that guard our system. Normally our cells recognize an intruder (such as bacterial or viral which are easy for the body to see) but cancer for some reason is able to avoid detection. Another way that this vitamin can help to prevent or at least slow down the tumor growth is that the vitamin C makes protein molecules which help to create immunoglobulins (anti bodies) which can recognize bad cells, combine with them and help the body identify and kill them.

It has been observed that when the immune system is suppressed as when immune suppressing drugs are given to help the body during the process of an organ transplant, certain cancers are more prevalent.

This in a small way shows that immune strengthening can help reduce the incidence of some cancers. Vitamin C given to cancer patients who are on a chemo therapy regimen can be helped as vitamin C can relieve some of the symptoms of chemo, making it tolerable and possibly reducing the amount of chemo needed for efficacy. Chemo destroys both the bad and healthy cells and vitamin C can help to repair the good cells damaged by chemo.

When you are on chemo, you won't be able to donate blood or donate any body organs. This is the frightening toxicity and devastating effects of this treatment. Therefore, anything that could help to reduce the severity of this toxin would be a great help.

In another study in Bangladesh, 1 gram of vitamin C was given intravenously for people below 30 years suffering from tetanus. The study showed they survived the illness while the control group subjects (that did not take the vitamin C) did not survive. It has been theorized that the over 30 year olds would have survived if they had been given more than 1 gram dose.

People suffering from diabetes show a significant improvement in glucose metabolism with vitamin C supplementation. It is very important for diabetics to take vitamin C as insulin injections lower vitamin C levels.

There are studies which also show the ability of vitamin C to regress colon polyps. It was found that there was a good recovery from toxic mushroom poisoning with the administration of vitamin C. All infections result in an increase of oxidative stress and this results in depletion of electrons from the molecules that are oxidized. Vitamin C donates an electron to aid in cell repair and therefore itself is used up. That's why adequate amounts must be taken.

In intensive care units, most patients are pre-scurvy as vitamin C is depleted due to the cells battle with the toxins. There is also evidence that using a vitamin C spray into the throat before smoking reduced the nicotine cravings, so this is great news if you are a smoker or trying to quit smoking.

Smokers would also benefit taking more vitamin C as 1 cigarette uses roughly 25 mg of this vitamin.

Those that have suffered from aneurysms have low vitamin C levels. In such cases, extra vitamin C will help. Vitamin C may help to cure swine flu. Alan Smith was in a coma and suffering from swine flu. Only after his loved ones begged the Doctors to administer intravenous C did he experience a total recovery. (If you have the time, check out the YouTube video of his very remarkable story).

The possibility of kidney stones is very rare and is more frequent in those with a low C level. A Harvard University study showed that vitamin C actually reduces kidney stone occurrence and helps to remove existing stones. Vitamin C has been shown to actually help prevent urinary tract infections. The only reference made to a possible negative effect is the increase of iron absorption which is contraindicated for those suffering from hemochromatosis (a rare disease where the body absorbs too much iron which can lead to damage of vital organs). Sugar also increases iron absorption. This is one of the reasons to watch your sugar if you have hemochromatosis. Interesting side note: pasteurization kills vitamin C. Babies fed with pasteurized milk were found to be deficient in vitamin C as the process of pasteurization kills the vitamin. New mothers should note this.

Stick with breast feeding if you can, as breast milk has adequate vitamin C content but only if the mother has sufficient vitamin C. In a recent study from the University of Copenhagen, maternal vitamin C deficiency could cause irreversible damage to the developing fetal brain. So expectant mothers should definitely supplement with C during pregnancy especially if they smoke which depletes this vitamin.

Researchers at Mount Sinai school of medicine have shown for the first time that large doses of oral vitamin C may help prevent osteoporosis by stimulating bone formation to protect the skeleton. This has profound implications for the elderly and women who have had their ovaries removed, as this procedure weakens the bones and effects bone density.

Remember that Billy goat I mentioned about earlier. Goats make up to 100 grams of vitamin C per day and rarely get sick. Dr. Frei has recently stated that "as more diseases are showing oxidation as their primary cause, vitamin C can help the body in the healing process as this vitamin is a very powerful anti-oxidant".

All infections promote oxidation. The more infection, the more antioxidants are needed to reduce oxidation and help in the healing process, vitamin C does just that. The natural sources of this vitamin are: guava (very high in C), leafy greens, kiwi, melons, oranges, red and green peppers and strawberries.

I still believe we all need more C than the diet can provide. I take 3 grams (3,000mg) per day of Ester C as it is buffered with calcium. Understand that too much circulating calcium can be a problem as it can get deposited in the arteries and heart. To be on the safe side, take sodium ascorbate which is vitamin C in powdered form ...simply mix with juice or water.

One other form of C is worth mentioning and that is Liposomal C, this is vitamin C that is combined with fat or more specifically phospholipid liposomes which are really tiny bubbles that form a protective barrier around their contents so that the nutrient will not degrade as from digestive juices, alkaline solutions, oxidation and general degradation. This helps the vitamin get into the blood and into the cell itself making this vitamin both fat and water soluble.

Bio-availability is the key and is simply the ability of the supplements to get to where you want them to be. Liposomal encapsulation technology allows this to happen. This technology keeps the nutrient safe until it reaches its intended target. Also, there are no additives like gelatin, binders or other fillers to dilute the substance. According to DR Thomas Levy this form of vitamin C is just as effective as intravenous C! This is ideally the form you should be taking.

Ideally you want to mix the forms of C so they can circulate in blood and in the cell itself for maximum benefit.

One last side note: if you were wondering about toxicity levels of C or taking too much, Professor Ian Brighthope M.D. Professor of nutritional and environmental medicine has experimented with over 200,000 mg of the vitamin in a 24 hour period with no adverse effects!

However, there is one note of caution from Dr. Mercola who has recently pointed to the fact that high doses of vitamin C could lower copper levels.

You may want to supplement with copper to keep your immune system working efficiently.

In summary, the uses of vitamin C are astonishing. Herpes Virus was stopped in vitro (in the test tube) as well as Polio virus! Acute viral hepatitis, and even rabies were inactivated in vitro. Cheap and powerful you really need to start taking vitamin C for a healthier and longer life.

"According to Dr. Andrew Saul, editor of the Orthomolecular Medicine News Service, "if everyone were to take 500 mg of vitamin C per day — the dose typically required to reach a healthy level of 80 µmol/L — an estimated 216,000 lives could be spared each year."

Vitamin E

Our next powerhouse vitamin is vitamin E. Vitamin E is a fat-soluble vitamin of which tocopherols and tocotrienols are composed. There are eight forms of vitamin E designated prefix as alpha, beta, gamma and delta. The most common form of E is A-tocopherol and has been studied more than others, especially the tocotrienols.

Vitamin E was discovered in 1922 by Herbert Evans and Katherine Bishop. When studying rats, they observed that the rats were not fertile even though they had adequate b and c vitamins. Only after feeding the rats with wheat germ, were they able to reproduce. The vitamin that was isolated from the wheat germ was vitamin E. It was named a-tocopherol from the Greek words meaning "to bear young." It was isolated by Gladys Emerson in 1935 and first synthesized by Paul Karrer in 1938.

The first therapeutic use was in 1938 by Widenbauer who treated premature newborns to correct growth failure. More than half were able to resume normal growth after administering vitamin E from wheat germ oil.

Vitamin E works in synergy with vitamin C. When vitamin E, a powerful antioxidant, becomes oxidized itself by scavenging free radicals, it becomes a tocopheroloxyl radical. It can become an active antioxidant again through reduction by other antioxidants, which is one of the reasons it is excellent when paired with vitamin C.

The alpha tocopherol is the most common form and helps with the following: heart disease, good for heart and blood vessels, high blood pressure, chest pain, atherosclerosis, cancer, arthritis, and may reduce the growth of cancer, particularly prostate and breast cancer.

This vitamin may also help prevent osteoarthritis, pain relief noted for the treatment of inflamed joints and the reduction of hot flashes in menopausal women.

This form of vitamin E may also help with the prevention of cataracts and macular degeneration. It also helps to control blood sugar, reduces LDL cholesterol and improves wound healing. It's great for diabetics in the reduction of inflammation, slows the progression of Parkinson's disease and improves athletic performance, as the vitamin can help by acting as a free radical scavenger. Free radicals are produced when your body is stressed by a vigorous workout.

Now we need to differentiate the different forms of E as this is critical in getting the full benefits from this remarkable antioxidant.
Scientists have found that different forms of E have different functions and benefits. Gamma tocopherol is another form of E and is also very important as it quenches the nitrogen free radical. This could benefit those suffering from prostate cancer and has been shown to slow the progression of prostate cancer

and improves those suffering from Alzheimer disease.

Vitamin E has also been effective in reducing fatty liver due to its anti-inflammatory nature. Another way that vitamin E can help is with reperfusion injury. Reperfusion (re-oxygenation) happens when blood is restored to an injured organ and is overwhelmed by the sudden influx causing oxidative tissue damage. Vitamin E can help to reduce this damage.

Next in the Vitamin E army are the little publicly known tocotrienols. These forms of the E vitamin are very powerful. In a recent study, they helped to reduce LDL in 4 to 10 weeks by 25%------- taking only 200 mg per day!

Arterial stiffness (arteriosclerosis) which contributes to high blood pressure as well as heart attack and stroke (also known as transient ischemic attack) was reduced and the blood vessels became more pliable.

Vitamin E aids in the fight against breast, prostate, skin and pancreatic cancer, as this vitamin sticks to the cancer sites and helps to kill them.

The natural sources of this vitamin are: avocado, almonds, cotton seed oil, grape seed oil, sunflower oil, and wheat germ oil as well as mackerel, salmon, tuna, sea weed (spirulina) and sunflower seeds.

The most effective form of tocotrienol is delta as this form is smaller than the other tocotrienols and can move around the cell quickly, bringing the benefits to all areas of the cell. The tocopherols will block the absorption of tocotrienols so it is best to not take these forms of E together or maybe avoid the tocopherols completely.

I take a minimum of 400 units of both forms daily. As this is a fat-soluble vitamin, I would not take more than 800 units per day.

Lipoic Acid

Next in our arsenal of supplements is "Alpha Lipoic Acid", also known as lipoic acid. You will find they are one and the same and are used interchangeably. Alpha lipoic acid was discovered in 1937, and in 1951 its structure was mapped out molecularly by biochemist Lester Reed.

You would need to consume seven pounds of spinach just to produce 1 mg of lipoic acid, something that is obviously not practical for most people.

Ala is unique in that it is a fat and water-soluble vitamin, and very easily crosses the blood brain barrier where it helps to protect brain tissue. Found in every cell in the body this Sulphur based powerhouse turns glucose (blood sugar) into energy. When ALa breaks down it becomes dihydrolipoic acid which itself is another powerful anti- oxidant, so you're really getting two for one and the ability of this nutrient to regenerate other antioxidants works well with the B vitamins which is the reason some call ALa the "network antioxidant".

Present in most foods, it is concentrated in, broccoli, kidney, liver, heart, spinach and yeast extract. There is some evidence that ALA can help to renew other antioxidants and even make them active again!

(Understand that Alpha lipoic acid is not that same as Alpha-linolenic acid, an Omega 3 fatty acids derived from plants similar to Omega 3 found in fish oil, which will be covered later). Ala helps increase the production of glutathione which helps the liver rid itself of toxic substances. Besides helping to utilize glucose, this compound also stimulates the regeneration of nerve fibers. Ala helps people with aids, Alzheimer's, cataracts, Parkinson's disease and stroke, as it detoxifies critical cellular areas. Ala may help diabetics as it improves glucose transport and also relieves peripheral neuropathy, and the pain, numbness and burning associated with it.

There are studies that suggest that Ala may help with cramps, burning, tremors and muscle weakness. Ala should be taken three times a day, 400 mg per dose. Take this supplement on an empty stomach 30 minutes before meals for maximum absorption.

The natural sources of this vitamin are broccoli, brewer's yeast, chard, kidney, heart and liver.

B Vitamins

In the 1940's, the importance of these vitamins was first recognized and for this reason flour, corn meal, and rice were fortified with B vitamins, restoring some of what was lost in milling, bleaching, and other processing.

Vitamin B1

Vitamin B1 was so named as it was the first B vitamin discovered. Thiamine or B1 is important for the nervous system and is often referred to as an anti-stress vitamin. It is so important for the nervous system that it was first called a-neurin for the devastating effects if it is not present in the diet. Thiamine helps to form the myelin sheath which wraps the nerves in a cocoon like cover to aid in the transmission of nerve impulses. This vitamin is also found in the skeletal muscle, kidney, heart and brain. Therefore, lack of this vitamin could result in muscle weakness and mental confusion

Thiamine has importance in turning food into energy by means of carbohydrate to glucose metabolism turning carbs into an energy source as in the formation of adenosine triphosphate or ATP which is an energy source used in every cell. Optimal levels of Thiamine are extremely important.

The big benefits of Thiamine are for muscle strength and mental acuity. Also benefits those with Leigh's disease, Crohn's, peripheral homeopathy, kidney disease, restless leg syndrome and reduction of heart failure as it helps to strengthen the heart muscle. Joint and rheumatoid arthritis, hip fractures, cervical cancer and athletic performance. (I.e. will help with sore muscles), were all improved with this supplement.

Anyone with diabetes should make sure you are getting adequate amounts of thiamine as this nutrient helps with the breakdown of sugar and carbohydrates. Also, many diabetics are thiamine deficient as their bodies do not absorb it normally and they tend to abnormally excrete more in the urine.

Those under a lot of stress and those using alcohol or if you consume lots of sugar would benefit from this nutrient. You should also understand that thiamine is continually excreted in the urine so deficiency is common if you are not getting enough from your diet.

I take B 100 complex 3 x a day which provides 100 mg of each B vitamin. Take your B vitamins with meals as this increase the absorption from 15% to 60%. (Very big difference when taken with meals).

The natural sources of B1 are yeast (nutritional), whole grains, flax, legumes, grains, brown rice, sunflower seeds, and eggs.

Vitamin B2

Next in the B line up is vitamin B2 or riboflavin which comes from ribose, a form of sugar from which the structure of this vitamin is formed. Flavin comes from the Latin "flavus" which means yellow, the color of this molecule, which also may impart a yellow hue to the user's urine.

Riboflavin is required for energy production in every cell of the body. This vitamin produces energy from carbohydrates, fats, and protein. Helps to produce glutathione, which is a very important and powerful antioxidant. It helps with liver detoxification and red blood cell production. Interestingly, this vitamin works synergistically with B6 and folic acid. Without B2, vitamin B6 is ineffective in some applications. Overall energy, healthy skin, liver, hair, muscle cramps, canker sores, memory loss, ulcer and the lining of the digestive tract---------- all showed improvement with this vitamin. B2 helps support adrenal function and also helps to maintain a healthy nervous system.

As far as the eyes are concerned, riboflavin helps to prevent cataracts and also helps to slow the progression of corneal ectasia which is a progressive thinning of the cornea. B2 is found in asparagus, milk, broccoli, spinach, eggs, almonds, yogurt cheese, whole grains, poultry, and lean meats. First used to help newborn with jaundice, later this vitamin was used to treat other illnesses.

In migraine treatment, 400 mg per day after 3 months reduced the recurrence of migraines by 50%. Aids in the production of red blood cells and helps get energy from fats, proteins, carbohydrates. There is an ongoing experimental use for Riboflavin and ultra violet light.

Scientists are finding that this combination of (B2) and ultra violet light is effective for inactivating pathogens in platelets and plasma viruses, bacteria and parasites. This study is ongoing but right now shows potential.

Vitamin B3 (Niacin)

Next in the B arsenal is B3 or niacin. It is so named as it was the 3rd B vitamin discovered. In 1873 Hugo Weidel first discovered this vitamin, which was later extracted by Casimir Funk in 1912. This vitamin was also called vitamin PP which stands for the pellagra preventive factor that is a therapeutic benefit which results from its use. From 1906 to 1940 3 million Americans had pellagra resulting in more than 300,000 deaths. Pellagra is a deficiency of niacin with symptoms ranging from indigestion, fatigue, canker sores and vomiting, to more severe symptoms such as thick scaly skin on exposure to sunlight, swollen mouth, red tongue, diarrhea, apathy and depression. Pellagra was caused by a poor diet of corn, molasses and salt pork.

Today the causes are no longer predominately from diet but are from digestive disorders and alcoholism. There is even some evidence that niacin can help to reduce drinking dependency in alcoholics and allow these individuals longer intervals without it.

Canadian soldiers who were imprisoned in Japanese war camps for extended periods of time showed severe malnutrition as they existed on 800 calories a day. Over 25,000 died in these prisons. Thousands more survived when they were given 3 grams of niacin per day. Niacin is used today in many third world countries for that very reason, to fight malnutrition. One proposed cause of malnutrition is undernourishment or the starvation of the cells---- B3 helps.

Those with Parkinson's disease were found to be brain deficient in Coq10 and NAD (Nicotinamide adenine dinucleotide) NAD is a co-enzyme in many biological oxidation reactions----B3 is a precursor to NAD.

Tuberculosis is a horrible disease caused by the bacterium (Mycobacterium tuberculosis). As much as one-third of the population may be infected with this disease which mainly affects the lungs but can also impact the pericardium in the heart muscle. Out of the 9.6 million cases of active TB, over 1.5 million people died, most of which occurred in developing countries. Niacin could help as the bacterium depletes the body of NAD. Niacin helps to generate more NAD, thus off- setting the deleterious effects of this disease.

Niacin helps recovery from brain damage. Yang and Adams injected nicotinamide in rats after study induced strokes---early injection of nicotinamide (form of niacin) reduced the number of necrotic neurons and "decreased the progression of neuro degenerative impairment caused by cerebral disease."

Related to this study is the conclusion that B3 may help protect against chemo-brain forgetfulness, confusion and lack of focus, which is hopeful news for those undergoing chemo-therapy. Dr Hoffer a prominent B3 research specialist, reported that a 60-year-old stroke victim showed improved memory and sense of well-being when treated with supplemental niacin.

Niacin is closely related to nicotine (it is an analogue) which means that they are very similar chemically and therefore taking niacin may help those trying to quit smoking. If you are a smoker and trying to quit, niacin may help you.

One of the current uses of niacin is for its ability to lower total serum cholesterol and specifically to raise HDL as well as lower LDL and lower total cholesterol. According to Dr. Steven Nissen president of the American College of Cardiology" niacin is really it, nothing else is as effective in lowering cholesterol levels". As discussed, earlier NAD is one of the most important co-enzymes in the body and helps in the repair of DNA.

Niacin is also important in the catabolism (the breaking down of complex molecules for releasing energy) or in providing smaller molecular units to build up organs or tissues of fat, carbohydrates and protein. Niacin produces anti-inflammatory effects in brain tissue, GI tract and skin as well as improving the vascular system. Niacin lessens neuro-inflammation and for this reason may be effective for MS and Parkinson's disease as this nutrient aids in repair of DNA and in the removal of toxins from the body.

Niacin has also been used to reduce injury in the brain after strokes. In a study by Yang and co-workers after induced strokes in animals found that nicotinamide (niacin amide) could save injured cells within the ischemic area. (restriction in blood supply to tissues).

In another study, people taking niacin (B3) and riboflavin (B2) had fewer cataracts than those subjects not taking these nutrients. In fact, another case-controlled study showed that an increase of only 6.2 mg of niacin resulted in a 40% decrease of oral (mouth) pharyngeal (throat) and esophageal cancers. This study was conducted in Italy and Switzerland. (Negri E, Franceshi S, Bosetti C,et.al. Pub Med).

In a study by Jacobsen and Jacobsen, cells were given niacin and then exposed to cancer. The cancer developed at a rate of only 1/10th of the rate in the same cells not given niacin, so there is reason to believe it can act as a shield protecting the exposed cells.

Niacin is also a help in those undergoing chemo therapy. A study by Bartheman, Jacobs, and Korkland showed benefits of niacin against the damaging effects of chemo-therapy. Dr. Abram Hoffer was a psychiatrist that treated schizophrenics with 1000 mg niacin three times daily and had lots of success using this vitamin.

The premise is based on the fact that when adrenaline oxidizes it becomes adrenochrome.

Adrenochrome is a hallucinogen and it is hypothesized that this by-product causes the visual disturbances experienced by these patients. Niacinamide (a form of niacin) is capable of blocking the conversion of adrenaline to adrenochrome.

Dr Hoffer was also able to terminate LSD reactions as LSD interferes with the synapses between nerves. Skin disorders such as acne, epidermolysis bullosa (a rare genetic disease) All improved with the administering of niacin.

Professor Darmian discovered that niacinamide was a better sunscreen protector than common sunscreens. Jacobsen and Jacobsen believe that niacin which converts to NAD (nicotinamide adenine dinucleotide) prevents processes that lead to cancer. In the National Coronary Drug study, niacin decreased the death rate from our number two (presently) and looks like it may become our number one killer----- cancer.

In the United States 30,000 kidney transplants are performed yearly. Over 100,000 people are on waiting lists for kidney transplants so anything that can protect your kidney is extremely valuable to you. Niacinamide can help to protect your kidney tissue. As far as toxicity is concerned niacin and its derivatives increase liver function, this does not indicate a liver pathology.

Always check with your doctor before starting a supplement regimen. In rare instances some individuals may not tolerate niacin well. The one form of niacin that should be avoided is time release. There have been negative liver side effects with this form of the vitamin. The newest and most powerful form of niacin is nicotinamide riboside. This is a new and more potent version of niacin.

In 2013 Dr David Sinclair of Harvard medical school conducted a series of experiments using nicotinamide riboside on mice. The results were amazing: in 2-year-old mouse cells after treatment with nicotinamide riboside their cell age decreased from being 2 years old to 6 months! Results included an increase in energy and elevated mood. Overall a younger more vital cell emerged.

These results if translated to a human model would result in increased metabolism, mental clarity, reduced risk of heart disease, cancer and Alzheimer's. Nicotinamide ribosome enhances communication among cells increasing cellular energy and metabolism in the process. This unique form of niacin prevents DNA damage and tumor formation also helps to reduce skeletal muscle aging and could be useful in Parkinson's disease.

The natural sources of vitamin B3 are brewer's yeast, almonds, wheat germ, organ meats, whole grains, wild rice, mushrooms, soybeans, milk, yogurt, eggs, broccoli, and spinach.

The next B vitamin is B5 or pantothenic acid discovered by American bio chemist Dr. Roger Williams, Ph.D. chemistry. Using yeast cultures isolated pantothenic acid later concentrated folic acid and named it also. Pantothen in Greek means "from all sides" which is appropriate as small amounts of this vitamin are found in virtually all foods.

This water-soluble vitamin is critical for health. This nutrient, like all B vitamins helps to convert fat, carbohydrates and protein into energy. B5 is a precursor to Coenzyme A (CoA). This is an essential co enzyme in a multitude of biochemical reactions that are essential for life. Coenzyme A and its derivatives help to generate energy from fats, carbohydrates and proteins. Coenzyme A is also involved in the synthesis of cholesterol, fats, steroid hormones, vitamins A and D, acetylcholine (neurotransmitter), melatonin and for the essential component of hemoglobin. In addition, liver metabolism of drugs and toxins requires CoA. There is an improvement in skin conditions with this nutrient as well as improvement in wound healing.

One thing to understand is that B 5 helps in the synthesis of cholesterol (cholesterol is not a bad thing although the LDL form is conducive to atherosclerosis as it can accumulate in the arteries and veins). Cholesterol is critical for health as the cells need it in the cell membrane. It is essentially like glue that keeps the cells structurally sound. Cholesterol is also needed for production of hormones. Some people taking cholesterol lowering medication suffer from actual muscle tissue loss. So if you can, try to lower your cholesterol naturally through diet, exercise and of course proper supplementation.

Pantothenic acid has been linked to possible improvements for the following conditions: acne, alcoholism, baldness, asthma, ADHD (attention deficit hyperactivity disorder), autism, arthritis, burning feet syndrome, yeast infections, heart failure, carpal tunnel syndrome, gray hair, headache, low blood sugar, insomnia, MS, MD, muscle cramps, osteoarthritis, rheumatoid arthritis, Parkinson's, enlarged prostate, shingles, skin disorders chronic fatigue syndrome, dizziness, eczema, insect stings and poison ivy!

More studies are needed to show a definite efficacy from these conditions but the early results are very encouraging. This vitamin along with all the B vitamins should be taken 3 times a day as they are water soluble. True to its name, this vitamin is found in small amounts in virtually all foods. Such as mushrooms, avocados, sweet potato, whole grains, legumes, meat, eggs and yogurt. I take a B 100 complex 3 times a day.

Vitamin B6

Next in the vitamin B arsenal is B6 or pyridoxine. In 1934 Hungarian Dr. Paul György discovered that this chemical cured skin disease in rats. He called it B 6. In 1938 Samuel Lepkovsky isolated B 6 from rice bran and in 1945 Snell discovered two forms of this vitamin: pyridoxine and pyridoxal. So named as it is structurally similar to pyridine. There are actually eight forms of this vitamin but the two most common forms, the pyridoxine and pyridoxal. There is a metabolically active form called pyridoxal 5 phosphate or P-5-P which is readily available at most vitamin stores.

The function and purpose of this vitamin B as well as the B complex is in energy production. In particular B6 is involved in macronutrient metabolism.

Nutrients are needed for growth and again the main nutrients are carbohydrates, fats and proteins. Macro means large so these nutrients and the B complex vitamins of which B6 is a component are needed to metabolize these macro nutrients. B6 is involved in the formation of myelin which is the protective protein layer that encapsulates the nerve cells.

Dopamine, epinephrine, nor-epinephrine and serotonin are necessary for the transmission of nerve signals in the brain. These help in facilitating the speed and integrity of the nerve impulses and aid in their communications by helping the signal cross from the synapse of the neuron to the target receptor. Also aids in the synthesis of serotonin, dopamine, epinephrine and GABA (Gamma-Amino butyric acid) an inhibitory neuro transmitter which helps to reduce neuronal excitability in the central nervous system. The other neurotransmitter synthesized by B6 is histamine which is yet another neuro transmitter which aids the body by vasodilation, recruiting more white blood cells to the area of infection and also by creating a fluid wash to remove toxins from insect bites or any poisonous agent.

Essentially the B vitamins are vitally important to the health of our nervous system and B6 should be taken along with all the other B vitamins to ensure the integrity of the central nervous system.

Cooking and storage can destroy B6 but it is unlikely that you have a deficiency of this vitamin unless you are elderly, alcoholic, or have HIV, liver disease or rheumatoid, arthritis. B6 is found in grains, pork, turkey, beef, bananas, chick peas, and pistachios.

This vitamin is beneficial for carpal tunnel syndrome, nausea and vomiting during pregnancy and in a recent study has showed promise in the reduction of colon cancer. Over 100 maladies may be helped with B6 as well as heart disease, PMS and may even help prevent kidney stones.

The amino acid homo cysteine is a risk factor for heart disease... B6 can help to lower homocysteine levels. Understand too that certain food dyes and yellow #5 and certain medications can interfere with vitamin B6 absorption. So you may want to avoid these additives and food dyes in order to gain maximum absorption. Again, this vitamin should be taken along with a B complex for maximum benefit.

Vitamin B7 (Biotin)

Next in the B complex arsenal is B7 or biotin. Surprisingly there are eight forms of this vitamin. We are concerned though with the most popular form which is D biotin. Biotin is also called vitamin H, the H stands for Haut and Haare, German for skin and hair. In 1916, W.G. Bateman found toxic levels from a large amount of raw egg whites. It wasn't until 1935 that Fritz Kögl and Paul Györy put a name to it.

Biotin is a coenzyme in the metabolism of fatty acids. This coenzyme speeds up the biological reactions helping the body to metabolize fats, carbohydrates and proteins. All organisms require biotin which can only be synthesized by plants, bacteria, algae and mold.

Biotin supports adrenal function, a healthy nervous system and helps blood glucose levels in type 11 diabetes. Adrenal function is extremely important. The adrenals are 2 reddish orange glands about the size of a grape that sit on the kidneys. As suggested by their name ad (for, at, upon) and renal (kidney).

The outer part is called the cortex which produces steroid hormones (cortisol and aldosterone and hormones that can be converted to testosterone).

Cortisol regulates metabolism and helps the body respond to stress. The hormone aldosterone helps the body by regulating blood pressure. The inner part is called the medulla and produces epinephrine and nor epinephrine commonly known as adrenaline and nor adrenaline. Adrenaline increases the heart rate and sends blood surging to the muscles and brain the clichéd fight or flight response we've all heard about. This helps in converting glycogen to glucose. This provides the energy boost needed in extreme stressful situations. Nor epinephrine on the other hand can cause vasoconstriction a narrowing of the blood vessels. Simply put, the adrenals produce hormones that regulate metabolism, immune system, blood pressure and sugar (glycogen to glucose) modulation.

There are some diseases which may be improved with supplementation i.e. Addison's (under production of cortisol) and Cushing's disease (over production of cortisol). Stress on the body can cause damage and this vitamin helps in some ways to lessen the severity of these effects. One interesting fact is that biotin cannot be absorbed through the skin or hair so hair and skin products containing this vitamin cannot be of help when applied externally. This vitamin may help to reduce nerve pain for those suffering from type 11 diabetes.

Although B7 deficiency is rare, low levels are found in alcoholics, burn victims, epileptics, and those pregnant and the elderly. All of whom may benefit from additional supplementation.

The natural sources of this vitamin are: Avocado, beef, broccoli, cauliflower, chicken, egg yolks, salmon and sardines. I take 5000mcg per day but this all depends on your unique bodily requirements, and your state of health.

Vitamin B9 (Folic Acid)

On to yet another important B vitamin: B9 or folic acid.

Named from Latin (folium) word for leaf. B9 is found in dark green leafy vegetables. We humans do not make folate and it is needed for DNA repair and also acts as a co- factor in various biological reactions. Initially it was used as a treatment for anemia as it helps to produce a healthy red blood count. It is important in cell division and growth. Especially needed during pregnancy and is one of the reasons that Doctors prescribe supplementing with this important B vitamin. It is used also to prevent neural tube defects and spinal bifida and is necessary for fertility in men and women.

Studies have shown a reduction in the risk of stroke. As evidenced by a reduction in pulse pressure. Can lessen likelihood of depression and age-related macular degeneration.

Folic acid occurs naturally in dark green leafy vegetables such as kale and spinach. It is also found in black beans, lentils, pintos, kidney beans, citrus like oranges, peaches and avocados, beef and chicken. This vital B vitamin should be taken at least twice a day in a b complex formula.

Another vitally important B vitamin is B12, also called cobalamin (methyl cobalamin is the preferred form of B12).

Like the other B vitamins, it is water soluble, so taking it more than once a day is recommended. This vitamin is extremely important in brain and nervous system health. The original discovery related to pernicious anemia and the ability of this vitamin to prevent it by aiding in the formation of red blood cells.

B12 is the largest vitamin known and is not easily absorbed. This makes the bioavailability difficult.

Studies in Framingham Mass concluded that 1 in 4 adults were deficient in B12. In some people there is a shortage of intrinsic factor which is needed for the absorption of B12. Intrinsic factor binds to B12 molecule and together passes through the stomach to your small intestine. As we age our body makes less intrinsic factor, in particular the stomach lining produces less, therefore the elderly, vegetarians, heavy drinkers, smokers and those breast feeding all reduce intrinsic factor which in turn slows or prevents the absorption of B12. Medication as in stomach acid reflux reducers (PPI'S) also lessen intrinsic factor. Metformin which is often prescribed for type 11 diabetes also inhibits B12 absorption, for these reasons supplementation is advised.

Another benefit of B12 is that it may help to reduce homocysteine levels. Homocysteine is an amino acid found in the blood---meat is the most common source. High levels are associated with heart and blood vessel disease. B12 helps by converting carbohydrates to glucose i.e. energy production. Helps in reducing depression, stress, brain shrinkage, reduction in cholesterol levels and prevents against stroke and high blood pressure. Skin, hair and nails are also improved from this vitamin. There has also been evidence that breast, colon, and prostate cancer can be reduced with adequate amounts of B12. A lack of this vitamin may cause fatigue, depression, and poor memory.

Vegetarians especially should be supplementing as this vitamin is found primarily in fish, shellfish, meat, liver, poultry, eggs and milk. There are studies which show that chlorella and fresh water algae may be a source of biologically active B12....More study is needed. As far as supplementation is concerned, many health professionals recommend B12 spray under the tongue where there are a large number of capillaries which are very small and may make it easier to absorb. This could be a very effective way for this vitamin to reach the bloodstream. As far as dosage is concerned, I take B12 drops sublingually once a day. The B vitamins are water soluble so there is very little concern of toxicity as the body will remove any excess.

Choline is included here with the B vitamins even though it is not technically a B vitamin, it works with other B vitamins such as folic acid (B9) and cobalamin (B 12). Choline is important for brain and heart health as well as nervous system function. Vitamin B5 along with choline makes acetylcholine a chemical which facilitates the transmission of nerve impulses by improving the conditions at the synapse of the nerve allowing for a stronger and more robust signal. That's why the brain, nervous system, and memory are improved with this nutrient. Again, this works when choline is taken together with B5. Those with Parkinson's and Alzheimer's have tested low in acetylcholine in the brain. In addition, it is critical that newborns have adequate amounts of this nutrient to improve brain formation. The liver is also helped as choline helps to move fat out of the liver and into the rest of the body.

The source of choline is lecithin and this nutrient is found naturally in cabbage, cauliflower, chick peas, green beans, eggs, lentils and soybeans. I take 100 mg per day.

Fat Soluble Vitamins

Vitamin A

Our first fat soluble vitamin is vitamin A. There are 3 active forms of vitamin A: retinol, retinal, and retinoic acid. This vitamin is responsible for regulating the growth and specialization of virtually every cell. When there is a deficiency, there is a higher likelihood of birth defects. In addition, embryonic development is also affected. Vitamin A increases hemoglobin and increases the mobilization of iron from storage sites moving iron to red blood cells which carry oxygen in red blood cells.

Over nineteen million pregnant women worldwide are deficient in this important vitamin and roughly 50% suffer from night blindness. Roughly one hundred ninety million pre-school children have low serum retinol, 50% end up dying and for this reason WHO (world health organization) and UNICEF (United Nations children fund) distribute vitamin A to prevent child mortality.

Women who are HIV positive and low in vitamin A are 3 -4 times more likely to transmit the HIV to their children. Those with skin, breast, liver, colon and prostate cancer can lower their risk of dying by taking 2 doses of 200,000 IU of vitamin A, so you can see how powerful this vitamin is. Retinitis Pigmentosa is a disease which causes blindness and the administering of 5,000 IU daily can slow the progression of this disease.

It is always prudent to consult with your doctor before beginning any vitamin program. In the case of vitamin A, you could potentially get hyper - vitaminosis which is a toxicity you must avoid.

Vitamin A comes from two sources: preformed retinoid and pro-vitamin carotenoids. Retinoid, such as retinal and retinoic acid, is found in animal sources such as liver, beef, kidney, eggs, butter, and dairy products. Carotenoids, such as beta-carotene (which has the highest vitamin A activity), are found in plants such as dark or yellow vegetables and carrots.

Vitamin A has primary importance in the visual cycle. In the retina there are 2 types of light sensitive cells: rods and cones. Vitamin A helps as it is a component of rhodopsin, a light absorbing pigment in the retina. After absorbing a photon (particle of light), Trans -retinal (a form of vitamin A) is converted to all trans- retinol (another form of vitamin A).Transported across the interstitial (between) space to retinal pigment epithelial cells, thus completing the visual cycle as the nerve impulses are generated by the optic nerve to the visual cortex in the brain.

In those underdeveloped countries, vitamin A deficiency may lead to xerophthalmia (dry eye), night blindness and unfortunately even total blindness as well as skin disorders. There has been research that shows that there is a reduction in death from measles, improvement of immune system and even the prevention of some forms of cancer as we have mentioned earlier.

This vitamin is important. The RDA is 700 mcg for women and 900 mcg for men. Again, a blood test is advised to determine your vitamin A requirements.

Vitamin K

The Danish scientist Henrik Dam discovered Vitamin K in 1929. It was called vitamin K as the first letter of the German word Koagulation. He discovered that a diet without cholesterol also lowered the amount of vitamin K, and lead to hemorrhaging in the chickens who were his lab subjects. Giving the chickens extra cholesterol did not help until he added vitamin K----- this solved the problem.

Vitamin K produces blood clotting factors (prothrombin) which strengthen bones, capillaries and prevent calcification. If you have calcification you may want to supplement with this vitamin.

There are 3 forms of this vitamin: K1 (Phyllo Quinone), K2 (Mena Quinone), and K3 (Mena Dione). K1 helps bones absorb and store calcium. Studies have shown too that K1 may help to lower the risk of hip fracture. So, the elderly may also benefit from supplementation.

Vitamin K2 (Mena Quinone) is manufactured in the body by our own intestinal bacteria. Anti-biotics or even a poor bacterial gut balance prevents adequate absorption of this vitamin.

K3 is an artificial form of K vitamin and is water soluble which is easier to absorb. There are studies which, although not definitive, show that this vitamin may slow the growth of cancer. Newborns are given injections of vitamin K to prevent hemorrhage, and it is recommended for those suffering with Crohn's disease, colitis, or liver disease.

The recommended dose is 1 microgram for every 2 pounds of body weight. The average dosage is 65 micrograms for females and 80 micrograms for males. More than 100 micrograms could cause liver damage.

This vitamin is naturally found in green leafy vegetables such as: broccoli, cabbage, cauliflower, kale, soybeans, spinach and strawberries. Green tea also contains vitamin K. I take a super K supplement which contains all three forms of this vitamin by Life Extension once a day. They have some great supplements and should be considered in your search for quality vitamins.

Vitamin D

Vitamin D is the next important vitamin that we will learn about. As a matter of fact, this "vitamin" is not a vitamin at all but rather a steroid hormone produced by the body. As a fat-soluble vitamin / steroid you could over saturate your tissues and too much is not a good thing. It is also responsible for bone and teeth strength. D increases the flow of calcium into the blood stream and also pulls calcium from food. Osteomalacia which is a precursor to osteoporosis may be caused by a deficiency of vitamin D.

This hormone regulates the production of phosphorus and calcium in the body. There are 30,000 genes in your body and vitamin D affects nearly 10% or 3,000 of these genes. Cancer risk could be reduced by up to 60% if we had adequate levels of D in our system. Cancer of the lung, pancreas, and ovaries, prostate and skin could also be prevented.

There are two forms of vitamin D. There is D2 which is ergocalciferol. This form is broken down to potentially harmful elements, too much may be toxic.

D3 on the other hand is similar to the hormone produced when the body is exposed to sunlight (UVA) and (UVB) rays. This form (D3) is broken down to calcitriol which may be helpful in fighting cancer.

According to Dr. Holick: 32% of children and 50% of the general population is deficient in this hormone. This really is the result of the medical community and even the CDC recommending that we avoid sunlight exposure to reduce our cancer risk. As more and more people avoid sun exposure our bodies make less and less D3, resulting in a vitamin (hormone) deficiency.

The elderly are particularly vulnerable as they produce 30% less of this vitamin. Dark skin is another problem –the skin blocks the absorption of the sun's rays. Any ethnic group that has dark skin has this absorption difficulty and needs to spend even more time in the sun. Serotonin which is the body's natural ant-depressant is also reduced when there is less vitamin D being made. The lower your vitamin D level is the more depressed you may be. This is a simplified explanation for SAD (seasonal affective disorder) which occurs due to lack of sun exposure.

Fat absorbs and traps this vitamin, so if you are overweight you may also be contributing to a reduction in vitamin D levels. There are numerous studies that show that vitamin D lowers the incidence of colorectal, prostate and breast cancer. Further this vitamin/hormone helps in fighting infections, such as cold, flu and influenza. D3 also helps with cardiovascular disease, heart attack and stroke. One study even showing a 50% reduction in heart attack risk. DNA repair is also improved and the immune system is strengthened with this supplement.

In a recent Dr. Mercola newsletter, according to Time magazine:

"People who took daily or weekly vitamin D supplements were less likely to report acute respiratory infections, like influenza or the common cold, then those who did not.

For people with the most significant vitamin D deficiencies taking a supplement cut their risk of respiratory infection in half.

People with higher vitamin D levels also saw a small reduction in risk: 10 percent, which is about equal to the protective effect of the injectable flu vaccine, the researchers say"

Blood tests are readily available to determine your vitamin/hormone level of D. The ideal level should be 50-70 ng/ml. Juice, milk, cereal and fungus along with animal products will provide D, however the best way to get this vitamin/hormone is through natural exposure to the sun.

In ancient Greece and Arabia illness was treated with sunlight. Now the WHO (World Health Organization) and even the surgeon general have come out against this natural healer. Yes, over exposure is not a good thing but 15-20 minutes in the sunlight can produce more than adequate amounts of this vitamin/hormone and our skin gradually (one month's time) builds up a thicker layer to protect us.

Interestingly Herodotus, (6 BC) who studied skull remains, noted that there was a difference in the skull thickness between Egyptian and Persian skulls. The Egyptians shaved their heads and worshiped the sun, they had significantly thicker skull bones than the Persians who wore large hats, avoided sunlight and consequently had much thinner skull bones.

A study on Vitamin D and growth, showed that women who are exposed to sunlight and who consequently have higher vitamin D levels while pregnant, have children that are taller and have stronger bones, whereas women who shun the sunlight and do not take supplemental vitamin D have children with smaller bones and grow to be less tall adults than those children with better vitamin D levels. Doctors know this and vitamin D is one of the many supplements given to pregnant women.

Up until the 1950's sunlight was used to combat "diseases of darkness" ----tuberculosis and rickets. Dr. Niels Finsen in 1903 used sunlight magnified through quartz lenses to irradiate skin lesions known as lupus vulgaris.

As sunlight was not available year-round this Doctor created what is now known as phototherapy: using light to treat human ailments. The Nobel Prize was awarded to Adolf Windaus for his work in synthesizing vitamin D. UVB light from the sun leads to photosynthesis of vitamin D.

The importance of light as therapy was applied to coal miners and was very effective in increasing their energy levels. Light therapy was used to combat illness before the advent of anti-biotics. One Dr. Auguste Rollier was a helio-therapist, meaning he used the power of the sun to treat tuberculosis with great success. The Doctor does emphasize that the entire sunlight spectrum is needed not only for the healing properties of the sunlight but also for the protective components that are vital when using sunlight for therapy. Remember that this treatment relies on a gradual conditioning of the skin to sun exposure, and one month is considered an average time for melanin to saturate the keratinocytes and corneocyte skin layers in order to afford maximum protection----- a natural sunscreen.

Although improved, the sunscreens of today have a photon conversion rate of 80%, which means that they will produce reactive oxygen species, which is bad news for your cells resulting in oxidative damage.

Other Vitamins

Choline

Choline is being included with the B vitamins as it is water soluble and works in close harmony with the B complex of vitamins. Choline is not produced by the body and therefore is an essential nutrient. Fatty liver disease, neural tube defects and cholesterol buildup, may be prevented when there is adequate levels of this lipotropic.

Choline is important for processing fat, heart, brain health and central nervous system regeneration. Choline makes acetylcholine when paired with B5. This neurotransmitter is found in the synapse and is responsible for the nerve signaling as it transfers the signal across the synapse through this chemical "puddle." As an aid in transferring nerve signals it helps with memory loss and general central nervous system health.

Parkinson's disease is also being studied to see whether improvement is made with supplementation. Choline may help those patients with Alzheimer's disease as many of these patients have low levels of choline in the brain.

Choline helps to produce phosphatidylcholine, which moves fat from the liver to the rest of the body to create cell membranes of which these fats are composed of.

In Europe, Doctors treat hepatitis and liver damage with phosphatidylcholine with good results. Lecithin is the food source that produces choline and the natural sources are: cabbage, cauliflower, chick peas, eggs, green beans, lentils, liver, red meat, rice, soybeans and split peas. The RDA is 425 mg for women and 550 mg for men.

Inositol

Inositol is considered a water-soluble vitamin, also called B8. This not an essential vitamin as it can be synthesized from glucose by bacteria in the gut. This element is found in concentrated amounts in the heart, brain and lens of the eye. It is also important in hair growth and strength and also helps to re-distribute body fat.

Inositol works synergistically with choline... it is important for growth of cells, bone marrow and eye membrane health. Inositol is a fat emulsifier and helps to break down fat and reduces fatty build up in the liver and also prevents arteriosclerosis (hardening of the arteries). Inositol has a calming effect as it helps to produce serotonin and acetylcholine which helps in nerve transmission.

Twelve grams per day were used to treat depression and the patients did show marked improvement. The natural sources of this chemical are: beans, cantaloupe, chick peas, citrus, liver, oats, pork, rice, wheat germ and whole grains. I take 500 mg once a day.

Paba (Para- Amino Benzoic Acid)

Is a member of the B vitamins and is part of the folic acid molecule. Like inositol it is also made by our intestinal bacteria.

It is important for hair strength and growth, it is also an anti-inflammatory and as such may help with osteoarthritis, depression and fatigue. It helps to produce erythrocytes which are red blood cells which carry oxygen throughout the body.

PABA is an ingredient in sun screen as it protects against UVB rays from solar radiation preventing sun burn and skin cancer, reducing wrinkles and keeping the skin smooth.

PABA is found in eggs, brewer's yeast, liver, molasses, rice, wheat germ and whole grains.

There is no RDA so many Doctors recommend low doses such as 50-100mg, 3 times a day.

Amino Acids

The structural units that make up our proteins are the amino acids. There are over 22 amino acids. They are very important as they are precursors to neurotransmitters in the brain (essentially how we communicate). They are also the building blocks of the body and are responsible for forming muscles, organs, tissues, nails and hair from the more than 50,000 proteins they help to create.

They consist of essential (can't be synthesized by the body) and non-essential (those amino acids that are produced by the body in the liver).

Essential Amino Acids

Histidine

Histidine is an essential amino acid and as such has to be consumed in the diet or supplemented in order to get adequate amounts. It is integral in the formation of the myelin sheath which surrounds the nerve cells and protects them from damage. It regulates growth and aids in the formation of blood cells. Helps with wound healing and tissue regeneration, it has been associated with reduction of inflammation and may help those suffering from arthritis. This amino acid helps to relax blood vessels and helps in lowering blood pressure. Histidine also helps to detox the body by binding with heavy metals helping to remove them from the body. There is even evidence showing that histidine combined with zinc shortened the length of the common cold by over 3.6 days. This amino acid is found in brewer's yeast, peas, walnuts, wheat germ, and soy beans.

Isoleucine

Isoleucine along with leucine and valine is a branch chain amino acid. This amino is great for body builders as it increases energy and helps to rebuild muscle tissue especially after heavy exercise. Helps also in the regulation of blood sugar which s inflammatory when unregulated.

This amino can help to burn visceral fat (i.e. fat that is in the deeper layers of the body). Energy is then created when this amino converts to glucose. Helps with recovery after surgery as it aids in the healing of bones, skin, and muscle tissue. Natural sources of isoleucine are: nuts, seeds eggs, meat, fish, lentils and peas.

Valine

Next in the amino acid arsenal is Valine. It is included here (out of alphabetical order) because it is one of the three branch chain amino acids that work in synergy. Valine also repairs tissue, regulates blood sugar, stimulates the central nervous system and helps to remove excessive toxic nitrogen which in turn lessens damage to organs and liver for drugs and alcohol. Deficiencies in valine have been linked to nerve damage, as the myelin sheath which protects the nerves may become compromised. Valine is naturally found in meats, dairy, mushrooms, nuts and soy.

Lysine

Lysine is the next amino acid and has very strong anti-viral properties. It is recommended for cold sores and herpes and may be used along with vitamin C and flavonoids to help prevent outbreak of cold sores and a very painful disease called Shingles which has its origin in the herpes virus. Collagen and muscle protein are stimulated and cold sores and herpes heal faster when this amino is taken. The natural dietary sources of this amino are red meat, potatoes, soy, eggs, fish and lima beans. Large amounts of this amino acid should be taken only under a Doctor's supervision as is intensifies the effects of anti-biotic such as neomycin and streptomycin.

Methionine

Methionine is an amino acid that aids in fat metabolism. This amino contains sulfur which helps to produce glutathione, the body's natural anti-oxidant. Methionine also contributes to the production of cysteine and taurine as both contain sulfur. The importance of this amino cannot be over stated as it helps the liver process fats which could help in preventing a fatty liver. The glutathione which it helps to form can rid the liver of toxins. Glutathione is integral to producing creatine which gives muscles energy and helps the heart and circulatory system. You may have heard of the supplement SAME (S-adenosylmethionine). This is a variation of methionine and is good for arthritis and depression. The synergistic nature of many of these amino acids underscores their need to be taken together and in the right amounts as they are very important individually as well as collectively. It would be prudent to consult your doctor before starting any supplement regimen. The natural sources of methionine are: beans, eggs, lentils, garlic, onions, soybeans, seeds and yogurt.

Phenylalanine

Phenylalanine is next in the amino arsenal. Phenylalanine is essential for proper functioning of the central nervous system responsible for the creation of epinephrine, norepinephrine and dopamine, the three very important neuro-transmitters. This amino acid is capable of penetrating the blood brain barrier thus allowing a direct effect on the brain as well as the central nervous system. This amino can make you feel more alert and energetic and unlike coffee it will result in a smoother less jittery energy boost. There are three forms of phenylalanine: D- phenylalanine, L-phenylalanine and DL phenylalanine. D-phenylalanine may lessen pain and is used to reduce pain. L-phenylalanine is great for mental clarity and mood. DL phenylalanine is obviously a combination of the two and will help with both pain mitigation and improvement in mental state of mind. Parkinson's disease, and schizophrenia have been treated with this amino. People with high blood pressure and migraines should avoid this amino and foods which contain it as this could aggravate the condition. The natural sources of this essential amino are: dairy, vegetables, legumes, beef, pork, nuts, seeds and shellfish.

Threonine

The next essential amino is Threonine. This amino is essential in maintaining protein balance in the body. Heart, liver and central nervous system require this amino. The heart contains high levels of threonine, so for vegetarians and vegan's supplementation is recommended. Threonine helps to create glycine and serine which are important for collagen, elastin, and muscle tissue. Good also for bones and tooth enamel and may help with wound healing. This amino has been used in ALS patients as it increases the level of glycine which cannot be given directly as it does not enter the central nervous system. A 1992 study showed that giving 7.5 grams helped in decreasing muscle spasticity. This amino is naturally found in green leafy vegetables, dairy, mushrooms and the largest amount is found in red meat.

Tryptophan

Our last of the essential amino acids is Tryptophan. The most common form being L tryptophan. D tryptophan is rarer and seldom used. This amino acid helps to create proteins, niacin serotonin and melatonin. To create these, the amino also needs iron, riboflavin and B6. This is why it is important not to take amino acids or vitamins individually as they work in harmony to create many of the essentials that the body needs. This amino also helps with depression and promotes sleep as it produces serotonin and melatonin which aids in sleep, appetite and mood. The latest information I have is that this amino is not available right now as there was contamination in the manufacturing process. The illness eosinophilia myalgia or EMS which is a flu like neurological condition was linked to one Japanese manufacturer, Showa Denko. I would recommend that this amino be avoided at this time until an improved manufacturing process is implemented. The natural sources of this amino are meat, fish, poultry cheese beans and nuts.

Non-Essential Amino Acids

The non- essential amino acids (meaning they are produced in the body) are alanine, arginine, aspartic acid, carnitine, cysteine, GABA, glutamine, glutamic acid, glutathione, glycine, ornithine, proline, serine, taurine, and tyrosine.

Alanine

Alanine is an amino acid that helps to convert glucose to energy and eliminates toxins in the liver. During stressful physical activity the alanine helps to protect the cells. Nitrogen and glucose are regulated and normalized with this amino acid. There is a process called the alanine cycle which is critical for energy production as this amino takes the excess nitrogen, converts to urea and eliminates it. For diabetics this amino may help to prevent night time hypoglycemia as it aids in sugar regulation. Alanine is also necessary to produce the B vitamins particularly B5 (pantothenic acid) and B6 (pyridoxine). The prostate may also benefit as those suffering from BPH (benign prostate hyperplasia) which causes urinary discomfort, have benefited from taking a combination of alanine, glutamic acid and glycine. The natural sources of this amino are: meat, poultry, eggs, dairy, fish and even avocado.

Arginine

Arginine is our next amino acid. This amino boosts the immune system (increasing the output of T cells by stimulating the thymus gland) regulates hormones, blood sugar and improves circulation. Diseases such as atherosclerosis angina, claudication (difficulty in walking), coronary artery disease, ED and migraine. All may improve with supplementation. I did come across an incident where an individual with a broken leg taking 12 grams of arginine per day was able to speed her healing process and made her lose weight. This is one incident and may not be significant. The idea is that this amino is a very powerful healer of bones, wounds, and general illnesses as it stimulates the release of growth hormone. One thing to avoid is eating large amounts of sugar before bed time as the sugar will block the release of this important hormone. Metabolizing creatine and nitrogen, lessening body fat and even helping with arthritis are some of the many benefits of this amino acid. The foods that contain arginine are: meat, peanuts, oats, walnut, wheat germ, and soybeans. You still may benefit from supplementation if you are recovering from an illness or healing broken bones or even suffering from arthritis. The increased blood flow will help in all of these conditions. This amino is contraindicated in herpes and schizophrenia and may actually make them worse. Always consult a physician if you are on medication of any kind.

Aspartic Acid

Aspartic acid or L aspartate is an amino that is used to combat fatigue, depression and even helps to produce energy. This production of energy is accomplished by moving NADH (nicotinamide adenine dinucleotide) into the mitochondria, generating ATP (adenosine triphosphate). This cycling creates energy as it is focused in the mitochondria which are the energy producing cells of the body. This process increases mental alertness, endurance and overall energy. The natural sources of this amino are: dairy, beef, molasses, sugar cane and poultry.

Carnitine

Carnitine is our next amino acid. This amino gets its name from where it was first discovered--- in meat. The Latin word for meat is carne. Carnitine or L carnitine carries fatty acids into the mitochondria, there converting these fatty acids into energy. Those with heart ailments or heart failure may find help with this amino. Studies have shown that carnitine may help with chronic fatigue syndrome, Alzheimer's, and depression. The decrease of LDL (bad cholesterol) and the increase of HDL (good cholesterol) have also been observed. Carnitine and its variation called acetyl L-carnitine is excellent for heart health and memory improvement as this form of carnitine produces acetylcholine which helps with memory loss. Vegetarians and vegans should consider supplementation as large amounts are not found in vegetables. The natural sources are: dairy, meat, fish and poultry.

Carnosine

Carnosine is quite different in its benefits. Many vitamins are considered anti-oxidants meaning that they help to reduce oxidation which can cause free radical damage to the body. A dangerous by-product of sugar is called glycation which is also a free radical and can further damage the body. Carnosine or L Carnosine can slow the process of glycation and extend the life of human cells. Toxic heavy metals have been linked to a number of diseases, namely Parkinson's, Alzheimer's, autism and dementia. Carnosine may help in chelation, a process whereby these toxic metals can be bound and excreted from the body. L Carnosine cream can improve the tone and texture of the skin, so this is yet another benefit of this amino. One other form of this amino is N acetyl carnosine, which in several studies when used as eye drops helped to dissolve cataracts. If you have cataracts or are worried about developing them you may want to consider taking acetyl carnosine drops as a preventative.

Cysteine

Cysteine is the next amino soldier to fight the oxidation/glycation battle. This amino is a sulfur containing amino acid that helps with hair, skin and nails and in the integrity of collagen, which contributes to the health of the connective tissue. Glutathione is a major anti-oxidant that is created in part by cysteine and has as its major aid in de-toxifying the liver. Interestingly, cystine and cysteine mirror each other and are converted to each other chemically. Cysteine has been used to combat acetaminophen over dose, as it helps in the detoxification of the liver which is adversely affected by too much of this chemical. There is evidence that this amino may also help with rheumatoid arthritis, emphysema and bronchitis as it breaks down mucous. Homocysteine is the by -product that results in the breakdown of this amino, so it is necessary to take vitamin C, vitamin B6, B12 and folic acid to break down this oxidative by-product. You will see N acetyl cysteine as a common item in the cysteine family, this amino variation is more absorbable so you should use it when available. The natural sources of cysteine are: eggs, dairy, meat and whole grains.

Glutamic Acid

Glutamic acid or glutamate is another in the amino arsenal. This amino acid increases neuronal activity and facilitates the communication in the brain and spinal cord. This amino is converted into glutamine or gamma amino butyric acid (GABA). Glutamine is like gasoline or fuel for the brain it improves intelligence, fights fatigue, can control cravings for alcohol and helps schizophrenics. This amino helps to push potassium through the blood-brain-barrier. Like other amino acids it breaks down fats and sugars producing energy. Behavioral problems in children are said to improve as well as MS, ulcers and a form of hypoglycemia from the use of insulin for diabetics. This amino breaks down to Monosodium glutamate, so if you are allergic to MSG or have migraines stay away from this amino as well. Our most abundant and widely circulating amino acid is glutathione. This amino acid is also called a tri-peptide as it is made from cysteine, glutamic acid and glycine. Produced and stored in the liver this natural anti- oxidant can help your vision and general immune system. Although found throughout the body, large amounts are found in the intestinal tract and lungs. When the body is stressed, as it is when it has an illness, this amino helps by boosting the integrity and strength of red and white blood cells. The natural sources of this vitamin are:

fruit and vegetables, asparagus, avocado, broccoli, cabbage, cauliflower, cantaloupe, grapefruit, kale, orange, potato, spinach, strawberries, tomato, and watermelon, meat, eggs and wheat germ.

Glycine

The amino acid Glycine is important for our nervous system and energy production. Glycine, arginine and methionine are required to make creatine. Creatine helps to increase the muscle work load by increasing the ATP (adenosine triphosphate) cycle which is normally short and makes it of a longer duration so the muscles can work harder, and for a longer period of time. Collagen, which is a protein in the connective tissues such as bones, skin, and muscle is 1/3 glycine. The digestive system and the central nervous system also rely on glycine as a necessary component. Glycine lessens seizure activity, bi-polar depression and improves the symptoms in schizophrenia when added to the patient's current medication. Glycine is a sugar substitute and may also have a calming effect. Prostate health may also be improved (reduction in water retention) and cancer too could be helped as glycine inhibits angiogenesis which is a process whereby blood vessels are formed to feed the cancer cells. The natural sources of glycine are: beans, cheese, fish, meat and milk.

Ornithine

Ornithine: Next we will talk about the fat burning, muscle building amino Acid ornithine. Ornithine is often found together with arginine as they burn fat, build muscle and release growth hormone. Ornithine will release more growth hormone than arginine but they do use different mechanisms to do so. Liver detoxification is a benefit of ornithine as it helps the liver in removing toxic ammonia. Large amounts of ornithine (over 10 grams) have been reported to aid in wound healing, recovery from surgery bone healing and repairing skin after burns. The natural sources of ornithine are: dairy, eggs, fish and meat. Large amounts have not shown any adverse effects except for stomach upset.

Proline

Proline is our next non-essential amino acid. Proline aids in the production of collagen and cartilage. Collagen is essential for skin health, while cartilage ensures that your joints remain flexible acting as a cushion where the bones meet other bones to form these joints and keep them from abrading. This is a reason that chronic back pain and osteoarthritis may be improved with supplementation. Athletes or those engaging in strenuous exercise may exhaust this amino. Supplementation is again recommended Proline along with lysine may help to reduce the severity of herpes. However, be careful to not take too much of this amino as that could throw the citric acid cycle out of balance, making the kidneys and liver work harder to eliminate the resulting toxins. The natural sources of proline are dairy, eggs and meat. The central nervous system and brain relies on our next amino.

Serine

This amino is created by glycine so as you are learning about the amino acids you can see how related they are as they are all needed to create as well as support each other. However, this creation and support has to be in proper balance to reduce the likelihood of too many toxins being created and therefore making the liver and kidneys work a lot harder. Serine is responsible for healthy RNA and DNA production, muscle formation, immune system health and even the formation of the brain. Nerves and nerve conduction is also aided as this amino helps to produce the myelin sheath which protects nerves and aids in the transmission of nerve impulses. Serine moves to catalyze tryptophan which in turn creates serotonin a mood - altering brain chemical. A shortage of this amino may lead to depression and a weakened immune system as this amino acid aids in the absorption of creatine. The body uses B3, B6 and folic acid to make serine. The natural sources are: gluten, peanuts, soy and wheat.

Taurine

Taurine is a very important amino for heart health. This sulfur containing amino is made from methionine and cysteine. Heart, brain, and nervous system regulation are a part of this amino acids purpose. Taurine regulates potassium, magnesium, and sodium in blood and tissues, preventing heart attack, arrhythmia, and also metabolizing fats. In one study 10-20 grams of taurine per day reduced PAC's (premature atrial contractions) by 50% and prevented all PVC's (premature ventricular contractions) but did not stop pauses in the heart rhythm. After adding 4-6G of arginine remaining PAC's and pauses were stopped. Taurine may help some people by regulating the excitability of the myocardium. In some cases, taurine restored energy and endurance, it also quiets the activity of the sympathetic nervous system and lessens the release of epinephrine.

Arginine on the other hand is a precursor to NO (nitrous oxide) and may be able to restore sinus rhythm by stabilizing the sinus mode. Again, adding arginine with taurine successfully helped arrhythmias. Taurine stimulates the immune system, regulates insulin and may even help epileptics by reducing the amount and severity of seizures. The natural sources of taurine are: dairy, fish, meat and milk. The last but by no means least non-essential amino acid is Tyrosine.

Tyrosine

Tyrosine stimulates the nervous system, speeding up metabolism and regulating mood. Tyrosine and phenylalanine make epinephrine, dopamine and nor epinephrine. Three very important neuro-transmitters. Phenylalanine helps to produce tyrosine and tyrosine metabolizes phenylalanine. Tyrosine also helps with low libido, anxiety, depression, headaches, Parkinson's disease and may suppress appetite when 850 mg is taken before meals. Do not take this amino if you have high blood pressure or migraine headaches. The natural sources of this amino are: Almonds, avocados, bananas, beans, dairy and seeds. Next in our arsenal of health supplements are the minerals:

Minerals

Minerals are essential for optimal health and in many cases need to be supplemented, as getting these in adequate amounts just from your diet is very difficult. These important trace minerals work synergistically with vitamins to make anti-oxidant enzymes to fight free radical damage. Boron, calcium, chromium, copper, iron, magnesium, manganese, molybdenum, potassium, selenium and zinc. These minerals work synergistically with other vitamins and minerals enhancing their presence.

Boron

Boron is a trace mineral and knowledge is relatively sparse as this mineral has only been studied since the 1980's. What is known is that this mineral helps in the overall health and growth of the body. It is thought to aid in the absorption of calcium and magnesium. Boron improves calcium absorption and helps by increasing the strength and density of our bones preventing osteoporosis and arthritis. Studies have shown that Boron can also help reduce inflammation associated with rheumatoid arthritis. Boron seems improve attention and mental clarity. This mineral is found naturally in almonds, apples, avocado, beans, chick peas, dates, hazel nuts, lentils, peanut butter, dates, raisins and walnuts. Besides diet, make sure you are taking a good mineral supplement containing this very important but overlooked mineral.

Calcium

Calcium is our next very important mineral. For bone, teeth and body health as well as the prevention of osteoporosis. Calcium is vitally important. Almost 99% of calcium is in our bones and teeth and only 1% is in our blood but if the blood gets too low in calcium it steals what it needs from our bones so it is important to keep our levels from being too low. What you don't want is to have too high of a dose either, remember what was previously mentioned, magnesium and vitamin K are necessary to push the calcium into the bones and what you don't want is an excess of this mineral.

This excess could lead to calcification of the arteries (atherosclerosis) and calcification of the heart muscle itself that could result in heart failure. Besides being important for bone and teeth health calcium also strengthens our connective tissue and aids in the transmission of nerve impulses. As we age, we also lose bone density so if you are over 35 you will also need to supplement. Calcium is found in the following food items: Almonds, beans, Bok choy, cheese, chia seeds, eggs, kales, milk, oranges, oat meal, sea weed, sesame seeds, soy milk, tofu and lots of others. Try to avoid over eating the calcium rich foods (eggs, cheese, and milk) as they can and for many people do cause problems.

Chromium

Chromium is the next mineral or micro-nutrient. It has been reported that 90 % of the population is deficient in chromium. This mineral is helpful in insulin control and blood sugar modulation, as it helps to move glucose from the bloodstream to the body's cells. The metabolization of carbohydrates, fats and proteins for energy production. Other studies have shown chromium to lower LDL (bad) cholesterol and raise HDL (good) cholesterol. Blood pressure too may be lowered so this is yet another benefit. The immune system may also be strengthened from this mineral as it helps to increase or slow the loss of DHEA (dehydroepiandrosterone), a reported anti- aging hormone.

Also, for the aging population it may help to slow the loss of calcium which is obviously important for aging bones which are less dense and may show signs of osteoporosis. There is evidence that those individuals that are deficient in chromium have a higher risk of glaucoma. Antacids may interfere with absorption of chromium, so for those taking these medications supplementation is advised. The natural sources of chromium are: banana, broccoli, grape juice, green beans, mashed potatoes and turkey. Recommended daily requirement is 50-200 mg (micrograms).

Copper

Copper is the third most plentiful trace mineral in the body. The highest concentrations are found in the brain and the liver. This mineral is important for cardiovascular, (arrhythmia) skeletal and nervous system health. The nervous system is improved from the production of the myelin sheath around the nerves that aids in the strengthening of the electrical signals for a more robust nervous system. Super oxide dismutase is a very powerful anti-oxidant that copper helps to create. Copper also aids in wound healing and preventing the arteries from hardening, lowering cholesterol (LDL), preventing aortic aneurysms, and keeping fibers healthy by increasing elastin are other reasons why you need to make sure you have adequate amounts of this mineral. Copper keeps skin and hair healthy by producing melanin which gives hair its color some prematurely graying hair has been reversed with the use of this mineral. Copper helps to form collagen which improves connective tissue, bones and skin.

Copper also works with iron by producing hemoglobin which is needed for storage and release of iron, specifically red blood cells which carry oxygen to the cells. Copper is used to treat anemia, rheumatoid arthritis, osteoporosis, bone density and joint health. There is an old cure for rheumatoid arthritis and joint pain that requires the individual to wear a copper bracelet, as the copper potentially will be absorbed through the skin giving the benefits of this mineral. The natural sources of this mineral are: almonds, avocado, barely, bell pepper, beets, brazil nuts, eggplant, hazelnuts, kale, mushrooms, nuts(pumpkin, sesame, sunflower seeds), oysters, shellfish, peanuts, pineapple, pinto beans, quinoa, raspberries, spinach, strawberries, sweet potato and walnuts.

As we saw with other minerals, use of antacids interferes with absorption, so yes, supplementation is advised. Vitamin C and Zinc need to also be used to achieve the full benefits of this mineral. The RDA of this mineral is 900 mcg (microgram) for men and women over 18. The takeaway here is that you definitely need copper in your diet for all the above reasons, however supplementing with a full mineral multi is recommended so you don't take too much of any one mineral.

Iron

The most common deficient mineral in the world is iron.

Iron makes hemoglobin which carries oxygen throughout the body. Infants, teenage girls, menstruating women, as well as pregnant and nursing women may need to supplement to avoid anemia. Men over 50 should be careful to supplement as a toxic condition could develop. There is a dangerous condition called hemochromatosis where the body stores too much iron, individuals who have this condition need to be very careful with adding additional iron and even vitamin C which slows iron depletion. Iron is found naturally in the following foods: cheddar cheese, chick peas, egg yolks, lentils, nuts, organ meats, prune juice, spinach and whole grains. The best iron supplement for absorption is carbonyl iron. Other forms are ferrous fumarate, ferrous gluconate and ferrous sulfate. RDA varies, but the average is women over 51 --14 mg and men over 19-- 10 mg. The take away here is the obvious avoidance of anemia and the health of the oxygen rich red blood vessels.

Magnesium

The next super mineral is magnesium. It is a Greek word for a district in Thessaly called Magnesia. Nearly 68-80% of the population is deficient in magnesium. The average adult has 22 -26 grams of magnesium in the body----60% skeletal, 20% skeletal muscle, 19% intra- cellular, and 1% extra-cellular. It is the 11th most abundant element in the body and is vital to all cells. There are 3,751 magnesium binding sites on human proteins. This essential mineral is necessary for over 700-800 chemical, enzyme and catalytic reactions, including the production of ATP (adenosine triphosphate) which is the main source of energy in every cell of the body. Important for bones and teeth, bowel function, relaxation of blood vessels and regulation of blood sugar levels. It also aids in blood pressure regulation, helps to prevent cardiac arrest, heart attack, fibromyalgia, a-fib, type 2 diabetes, cardio vascular disease, aging and all-cause mortality.

In a coronary care study 24 grams were given IV to patients who were then followed for 5 years and there was an overall decrease in all-cause mortality. There is no study that I have found that after one IV treatment would reduce mortality this dramatically in a 5 year follow up. Glutathione which is the body's super antioxidant is synthesized from magnesium so the importance of this mineral keeps surfacing.

It is a creator of protein, muscle movement, and the regulation of the central nervous system, as it is a precursor to neurotransmitters such as serotonin. It also plays an integral role in the formation of DNA and RNA the essential building blocks of the body's molecular structure. The creation of ATP (adenosine triphosphate) which is the body's energy source is also dependent on this mineral.

The highest concentration of magnesium in the body is found in the heart -if the concentration is too low then the heart can't function properly. Magnesium also helps in the regulation of calcium, when there is too much calcium, calcification, heel spurs, kidney stones and atherosclerosis is allowed to flourish. Calcium is excitatory to the neurological systems in the body, again too much calcium is really not a good thing and everybody could benefit by watching their calcium intake.

Magnesium is a calcium regulator and relaxes muscle whereas calcium contracts it. Magnesium is also necessary for calcium absorption as well as the uptake of potassium and the conversion of vitamin D 3 into its active and useable form. An interesting fact is that the Japanese who take less calcium but more magnesium have a lower incidence of osteoporosis. Deficiency of magnesium may lead to numbness, tingling, muscle cramps, contractions, coronary spasms, and abnormal heart rhythms.

In 1618 a farmer at Epsom in England discovered that his cows would not drink the water due to the bitter taste. However, it was also noticed that the water seemed to heal abrasions, scratches and skin rashes. This was the origin of the therapeutic use of Epsom salt (magnesium sulfate).

The following are some of the unique properties of magnesium use. IV magnesium is recommended for ventricular arrhythmia (specific heart rhythm abnormality). It is also used for the reduction of PMS symptoms as it helps to reduce water retention and bloating, helps in the relief and prevention of migraine headaches, aids in the absorption of sugar from the blood which can help to reduce insulin resistance. Fights inflammation which helps with general fitness and health and also could help with those suffering from arthritis as inflammation is the chief cause of this illness. Magnesium may increase energy as it helps in the production of ATP which is our main energy source.

Sleep may also benefit, as this mineral aids in the production of serotonin (substance that helps to regulate nerve signals)...aids in sleep, mood, and depression and along with calcium, vitamin D, vitamin K can improve bone strength as magnesium helps to transport calcium and get it in to bone matter. Too much calcium and too much vitamin D can result in a depletion of magnesium as you are spreading the need for extra magnesium in converting D to active form and pushing the calcium into bone. (It has been recommended that you take no more than 2000 mg vitamin D per day).

There are many types of magnesium and the benefits are different depending on which form is being used. The following are some of the best forms:

Magnesium carbonate 45% magnesium.... has antacid properties.

Magnesium citrate has magnesium with citric acid, has laxative properties.

Magnesium chloride/magnesium/lactate has 12 % magnesium but is well absorbed.

Magnesium Glycinate / chelated form of magnesium, has a very high level of absorption, excellent for those trying to increase their levels of this mineral.

Magnesium oxide /non-chelated contains 60 % magnesium and may be beneficial for stool softening. This form is not well absorbed and should be avoided.

Magnesium sulfate/ magnesium/hydroxide is a laxative (milk of magnesia). Use with care.

Magnesium Taurate is magnesium and taurine (amino acid) has a calming effect on nervous system.

Magnesium citrate in powder form is great for mixing with juice and drinking throughout the day.

The latest version of magnesium is called magnesium Threonate which has the ability to be absorbed through the mitochondria. This could be the best one yet due to the heightened bio-availability.

There is one other magnesium product that is very interesting and one that I just started using. It is called re-mag and is a liquid form of this vitamin that is extremely tiny developed by Dr. Carolyn Dean M.D.N.D. it is "Pico" size which means it is one trillionth of a meter in size and for this reason can be easily pulled into the cells.

This new formulation should help to safely increase magnesium levels. Magnesium is not tested with a simple blood test as it is most prevalent in the cells. The one test that is recommended to check magnesium levels is RBC. This test can be ordered from request a test (go online for company website). Always check with your physician to be on the safe side. The good news about magnesium is you really can't over dose on this mineral. The most common complaint is the laxative effect that some people experience with the pill forms. Magnesium aspartate is chelated with aspartame which is a dangerous artificial sweetener and should be avoided.

The best dietary sources of magnesium are: green leafy vegetables, (spinach, swiss chard), beans, nuts, seeds, (almonds, pumpkin, sesame and sunflower) seaweed and spices such as coriander, almond milk, flax seed, whey and almond butter.

Manganese

Manganese is our next essential trace mineral that is critical for every life form. The brain and nervous system function properly in part because of manganese. From bone health, to sugar level control, a natural anti-inflammatory, manganese helps with any disease that has inflammation as its cause, such as one of the biggest diseases in the aging population----- arthritis. Those that suffer from this illness have low levels of SOD (superoxide dismutase,) this is the natural, very powerful, anti-oxidant that helps general body health and has as its component manganese.

There is another SOD that is formed from copper and zinc. It is currently thought that ALS (Lou Gehrig's disease) is the result of low levels of this form of super anti-oxidant. Therefore, you can see how important these minerals are. Helping to create essential enzymes that contribute to building bone as well as bone structure and bone metabolism. From the formation of connective tissues to calcium absorption to thyroid integrity and the proper functioning of sex hormones, Manganese is involved in all of these processes and also contributes to the metabolism of fats and carbohydrates. Roughly 35 % of the world population is deficient in manganese, due in large part to a poor diet. So supplementing with a balanced mineral distribution is essential.

So again, the benefits of manganese are:

Healthy bones- including improvement in the mineral density of the spinal column and the prevention of osteoporosis.

Blood sugar control - which is important for diabetics.

Epileptic seizures are in part the result of low levels of Manganese, these may be lessened.

Regulation of the body's metabolism including the metabolism of vitamins like vitamin E and B1, helps the brain, nervous system and even helps with digestion.

Thyroid health- an essential element called thyroxin, it is the most important hormone in the thyroid gland is in part composed of manganese.

Make sure you are getting enough without getting too much. A balanced mineral supplement is really all you need.

Molybdenum

Molybdenum is our next trace mineral. Discovered by Swedish scientist Carl Wilhelm Scheele in 1778 this trace element helps to perform some very important functions and is found in all tissues of the body, such as bones, liver, kidney and teeth. This mineral makes the enzyme xanthine oxidase, which helps in the metabolism of iron. Low levels may result in anemia and even tooth decay. Molybdenum helps to form or activate aldehyde oxidase which helps to detoxify acetaldehyde which is a toxic substance that may cause cancer. Asthma sufferers may benefit from molybdenum as this mineral converts sulfite, which some people are allergic to, into harmless sulfates which the body can easily tolerate. Sulfites may also cause itching hives and respiratory problems so the ability of this mineral to neutralize these sulfites is extremely important for some people. Molybdenum may also help with anemia as it helps to mobilize iron. Anemia can be a dangerous symptom of a more severe underlying illness, so a visit to the Doctor would be prudent. Molybdenum is found in dark green leafy vegetables, beans, liver, milk and peas. Again the take away here is that even though these are trace minerals they work to potentiate vitamins so they are needed. RDA is 150-500 micrograms.

Next in the trace mineral category is potassium.

Potassium

Potassium was first isolated from potash, that's where it got its name. All living cells need potassium for normal nerve transmission, muscle contraction, regulation of fluid flow throughout the body, blood pressure regulation and transmission of nutrients in and out of the cells. The ratio of sodium (which raises blood pressure) to potassium (which lowers blood pressure) is more important than the level of either mineral alone when it comes to developing heart disease.

This ratio of sodium to potassium across cell membranes is called the membrane potential. Almost like a battery it is used to power molecular devices within the cell and transmits signals for use by the neurons and muscle cells. This is a delicate balance that has to be maintained. The right amounts of sodium and potassium do just that. A recent study in the Archives of Internal Medicine followed 12,000 adults for a 15 year period.

The risk of dying from CHD or coronary heart disease was greater in people who had more sodium and less potassium then the other way around, even accounting for other factors such as weight, smoking and exercise, the sodium -to -potassium balance was most important and twice as many people died from this poor balance of potassium to sodium. This should be a good reminder to make sure you are getting adequate amounts of potassium and reducing your intake of sodium. Too much of a good thing is not good either. Too much potassium can result in hyperkalemia, (abnormally elevated potassium in the blood) this could be due to kidney failure or simply taking too much.

Be careful as this could result in palpitations, muscle numbness and even heart failure. Always strive for a balance in supplementation. If you have kidney disease or take ACE inhibitors or have heart disease or diabetes, you may want to watch your potassium levels as you may have either an impaired way to eliminate the excess potassium or take medication that can raise blood levels of this mineral. On the other side of this spectrum is too little potassium, which is called hypokalemia. Hypokalemia results in muscle weakness, fatigue and dangerous heart arrhythmias. The natural food sources for this mineral are: apricots, bananas, carrots, granola, mangos, melons, milk, oranges, peanut butter, potatoes, tomatoes and yogurt. RDA recommends 4700 milligrams daily intake. Talk to your Doctor as he can perform tests that will determine whether you have adequate amounts or need to supplement.

Selenium

Selenium is a very important trace mineral and the next in the mineral arsenal. Selenium comes from the Greek "Selene" which means moon, discovered in 1817 by chemists Jon's Berzelius and Johan Gann. Selenium in trace amounts is necessary for cell function. This mineral improves overall immune system strength, lessens heart disease, ensures healthy blood vessels and reduces likelihood of stroke. Selenium is incorporated into proteins such as seleno-proteins and is integral to creating glutathione, the bodies' ultimate anti-oxidant. Selenium works synergistically with vitamin E and has been called a chemo preventive in that it may help to slow the growth of cancer.

Although there are conflicting studies it is worth putting selenium in your arsenal as there are many other benefits, which include: the reduction in colorectal, lung and prostate cancer by 50% according to one 10 year study. The conclusion reached by the researchers suggested that selenium prevented blood vessels from forming to cancer cells thereby starving these cells. Those with HIV and Crohn's had low levels of this mineral. Hashimoto's disease is where the body attacks its own thyroid. Selenium is needed by the thyroid, so some doctors do recommend using it for this illness. Selenium has also been used to reduce mercury toxicity as it may help to remove it from your system.

Selenium is found naturally in soil and also in foods, such as beef, cod, mushrooms, poultry and walnuts. Too much selenium may lead to selenosis which could result in cirrhosis, fatigue and neurological damage. There are three different forms of selenium and their effectiveness depends on which one is used and what problems you are trying to remedy. The first is called sodium selenite-this form is a simple selenium salt and is used to bolster the immune system. Selenium methyl L-seleoncysteine, may trigger cancer cell death through a process known as apoptosis, where the cancer cells literally commit suicide. This form is effective against most cancers. Selenium from yeast is a general immune system stimulant and anti-oxidant. The RDA is no more than 400 mcg per day. I take one form of selenium, you may want to try other forms as they may be more effective depending on the condition you are trying to rectify.

Zinc

Zinc is the last mineral we will learn about. This is a very powerful immune strengthening mineral necessary to sustain life. Over 3000 proteins contain zinc and over 300 enzymes need zinc to function properly. Zinc is also needed for proper maintenance of vitamin E levels, absorption of vitamin A and the proper function of the immune system. There are between 2-4 grams of zinc in the human body. Zinc is found in the brain, muscles, bones, kidney and liver. The largest amounts of zinc are found in the eye (retina) and the prostate. Adequate amounts of this mineral are crucial for these organs to function.

Wreckage from the ancient Roman ship Relitto Del Pozzino (circa 140bc) contained the oldest known zinc pill (Zinc carbonates, hydrozincite and smithsonite). These zinc pills were used for sore eyes. The fact that a large concentration of zinc is found in the retina makes scientific sense to use zinc for eye health. Zinc helps to increase the effectiveness of vitamin A which helps vision. The fact that this was known at this ancient time is surprising. Zinc is stored in the brain and it is not surprising that zinc insufficiency in the developing fetus leads to stunted brain growth. Expectant mothers should take a good multi with plenty of zinc to ward off this potential defect.

In the adult brain zinc is stored in specific synaptic vesicles. The synapse is where nerve impulses cross a liquid pond to further communicate and send impulses to other areas of the body. Too much zinc can lead to neuro-excitability and has been called the brains dark horse as too much can act as a neuro toxin. Again, balance is the key with supplements. As too much of any of these supplements is not a good thing. There are several other areas that are worth mentioning. Zinc has been used to treat anorexia nervosa.......an eating disorder where the individual has severe caloric restrictions which can lead to death.

Adequate amounts of zinc decrease the appetite and make it easier for the person to have a healthier, normal appetite. Zinc is a very powerful anti-oxidant that helps to increase thymus gland functioning which helps to produce T cells which in turn boost the immune system. Immune system health as well as the reproductive and digestive systems are all helped by adequate zinc levels. Healthy skin, such as acne, burns, eczema, psoriasis, recovery from surgery, bone, hair and eye health (can decrease macular degeneration) growth hormone, prostate and thyroid-- all are improved with adequate amounts of zinc. There is some evidence that zinc may help to lessen the duration and severity of the common cold and flu, sore throat, canker sores, and tinnitus.

The natural sources of zinc are dark chocolate, fortified cereals, fruits, meats, (lean beef) mushrooms, and nuts, such as almonds, cashews, pecans, peanuts, pine nuts, pumpkin seeds, oysters, shellfish, spinach and squash. The different supplements are zinc acetate, zinc gluconate, zinc orotate, zinc oxide, and zinc pyrithione. Zinc acetate is good for skin, aging, muscle health and also helps to relieve cold symptoms. Zinc gluconate is used primarily for maintaining the bodies zinc levels, but is not recommended to take with blood thinners (Coumadin), or antibiotics such as tetracycline and ciprofloxacin. There are some Doctors who maintain that this form of zinc is not readily absorbed. They along with others really like the absorbability of our next zinc form... which is zinc orotate. This claim about absorption is based on the fact that this form of zinc is neutrally charged and easier to get into cells. Zinc oxide is used in topical ointments for the treatment of burns, irritation and may even help to heal the wounds of surgeries. Zinc pyrithione is used in shampoos to prevent dandruff. As we said before, zinc does help skin and scalp.

The RDA of this mineral is 15 mg for men and 12 mg for women. It is advised that you not exceed 40 mg per day as copper consumption will be compromised. Too much zinc can trap this mineral and prevent absorption.

These next supplements are very important and are right now in the public's eye as they have some very substantial benefits.

Honorable Mentions Supplements

Coq10

Coq10, Curcumin, Omega3's (fish oil), and Resveratrol. Coenzyme q 10 or coq10 is a coenzyme which helps enzymes and can also function as an anti-oxidant. Coq10 is a fat-soluble supplement otherwise known as ubiquinol. This supplement is from a class of compounds known as quinines, discovered in 1957 by a researcher at the University of Wisconsin and later synthesized by scientists at Merk.

Coq10 is found in every cell of the body and is actually made by your body but as we age this production lessens. Coq10 is found in the energy producing cells of the body known as the mitochondria. Coq10 is involved in the production of adenosine triphosphate (ATP) which is a cellular energy component. The tremendous energy needed by the heart makes this supplement necessary for maximum heart health. In 1964 Japanese Doctors touted the benefits of this supplement for congestive heart failure as this helps the heart by increasing the energy of the heart muscle cells and by acting as an anti- oxidant to quench the free radicals which can damage this muscle.

Many people are now taking statins to help lower cholesterol and when these drugs are taken Coq10 is decreased, therefore it makes sense to take a Coq10 supplement especially if you are on statin medications. Biochemist, Karl Folkers PhD discovered the role of Coq10 in fighting heart disease. Over 70% of his heart patients showed improvement after taking this supplement. In 1961 researchers noticed that people with cancer had low levels of Coq10. These cancers included: breast, colon, kidney, lung, pancreas and prostate cancer. One study with 41 women who had breast cancer --- showed that all women improved by adding Coq10.After several weeks of use, Coq10 may even lower blood pressure and can help those with Alzheimer's as it aids in strengthening circulation.

There are studies also which show an improvement in those suffering from migraine headaches. Coq10 works best with vitamin E and DHLA (di hydro lipoic acid.) As this supplement helps with cellular healing it could help to improve gum disease by aiding in the body's ability to restore the gum tissue. The natural sources of Coq10 are: beef, broccoli, (dark leafy greens) chicken, nuts, pork and shellfish. It is always desirable to get your supplements from natural sources but in this case, you only get 2-5 mg, which is not enough. There are two forms of this supplement. Ubiquinol is the active form and ubiquinone is the oxidized form. Most supplements contain both. It is more ideal to take ubiquinol which is the active form that the body creates when Coq10 (ubiquinone) is taken, so ubiquinol is the most potent form and should be used when possible.

As there is no RDA for this supplement it is generally recommended by Doctors to take 90-120mg per day. Up to 3600 mg have been taken with no adverse effects. However, 100mg per day should be sufficient and as this is a fat-soluble supplement it should be taken with meals containing fat for maximum absorption.

Curcumin

The next supplement that is very popular and very powerful is the bright yellow spice turmeric and the active extracted substance called curcumin.

Curcumin is a curcuminoid from the ginger family and has been used in India for 1000's of years. Curcumin is a natural anti-inflammatory, and works by blocking Nf-kB. (Nuclear factor kappa-light-chain-enhancer of activated B cells). NF-Kb plays a role in the immune response to infection and is linked in a complex array that involves inflammation, and progression and promotion of some cancers.

Curcumin helps to block this cascade of events by blocking NFkB at the molecular level. Curcumin increases the anti-oxidant capacity of the body, blocks free radicals and even stimulates the bodies own ant-oxidant enzymes. Curcumin also boosts BDNF (brain derived neurotrophic factor) which helps to create new neuronal connections. Lowers the risk of brain diseases and improves brain function. Low levels of BDNF has been linked to depression and Alzheimer's, so there may be help for those suffering these illnesses. Since curcumin crosses the blood brain barrier it may be a help to Alzheimer's sufferers as inflammation and oxidative damage is reduced. Those with Alzheimer's also have a buildup of protein tangles, called amyloid plaques, curcumin can help to clear these plaques. Circulation is also improved as curcumin helps the endothelium which is the lining of the blood vessels. Arthritis involves inflammation of the joints and curcumin can reduce inflammation and has shown to offer some relief from this condition.

Depression is another condition which can be improved with curcumin. A recent study had patients take Prozac and curcumin and some took both curcumin and Prozac. After 6 weeks there was improvement and the best results were from those patients who took both curcumin and Prozac. More research is needed but the results were excellent. The positive results may be the result of curcumin's ability to boost the brain neurotransmitters such as serotonin and dopamine. In a recent study 44 men with lesions in their colon took 4 grams of curcumin per day for 30 days and this regimen reduced the number of lesions by 40%. Curcumin helps to reduce angiogenesis, a process which grows new blood vessels in tumors. Metastasis (cancer spreading) is also reduced when this natural spice is used.

This cancer fighter really needs to be in your supplement arsenal. Curcumin is poorly absorbed and there has been evidence that black pepper enhances absorption by as much as 2000%. So you would be advised to find curcumin supplements with this combination of black pepper or bioperine which is black pepper extract. Experiment and take throughout the day. There is no known toxicity, so that should not be a concern. Remember everybody is different and you may need to use more to get the desired effect.

Fish Oil

Next are the often spoken of Omega 3's.EPA (eicosapentaenoic acid) and DHA (docosahexaenoic acid). EPA is an Omega 3 fatty acid that is a precursor to chemicals involved in blood clotting and inflammation. DHA is an Omega 3 fatty acid that is a major component of the human retina, sperm and cerebral cortex.

Mother Nature knows the importance of Omega 3's as breast milk contains a high percentage of this fatty acid.

The following list of benefits is really overwhelming. Depression. DHA and EPA may help to fight depression. Researcher Dr. Andrew Stoll concluded that since the cell membranes are partially composed of Omega 3's, increased blood levels allow serotonin to circulate freely delivering this natural chemical anti-depressant to the body's cells.

The Mayo Clinic and the American Heart Association recommend fish oil to reduce cholesterol and lower triglyceride levels. Inflammation is reduced when fish oil is used and this may help the thyroid and diseases such as lupus. Inflammation is also implicated in osteoarthritis and rheumatoid arthritis. The Albany medical college used fish oil to reduce the pain of rheumatoid arthritis and did have positive results. Weight loss is another benefit from this amazing oil. The University of Georgia in the Journal of Nutrition found that fish oil prevents pre-fat cells from becoming fat cells and lets them die, how this is accomplished is not fully understood but is another of many reasons to supplement.

Skin

EPA in fish oil is also good for the skin. In the Journal of Lipid research, oil production, increased hydration, less acne, fewer wrinkles and even UVA sun protection were some of the benefits of this oil. If all this weren't enough Dr. Patrick McGorry in Australia, found a correlation between fish oil levels and the development of schizophrenia. In his study he found that only 3% of those treated with fish oil went on to develop schizophrenia whereas 28% of those taking a placebo developed this disease. Pregnant women taking fish oil gave birth to children with higher IQ's, fewer learning disorders and were less likely to develop mental retardation.

Mothers were also helped as Omega 3's reduced the postpartum depression, possibly due to the increase in circulation of serotonin and mothers were also able to continue breast feeding, something that has to be stopped when drugs are prescribed. Studies in Australia have shown that adults who take Omega 3's are less likely to develop macular degeneration due to the visual improvement when Omega's are used. Alzheimer's patients may be helped as this supplement helps to fight amyloid plaques which build up and compromise neuronal signaling. Studies have shown some promise in Omega 3's ability to slow the tumor growth rate in breast cancer. If all this weren't enough to convince anyone to add this supplement the University of Maryland medical center studied the effect of Omega 3's on peptic ulcer healing and the results were encouraging.

Ulcers in the colon and intestines were also improved with this supplement. Dr. Edward Hallowell center for ADHD (attention deficit hyperactive disorder) have achieved good results with this supplement as children with ADHD have lower blood levels of Omega 3's. As this oil curbs inflammation, it will help with blood vessel health which is integral to heart health. There is evidence that high doses 3-4000mg helps to curb abnormal heart rhythms (arrhythmias). The natural source of omega 3's are obviously, fish. DHA and EPA are the best forms of fish oil and they come from... you guessed it... fish. Fresh Salmon is best ...avoid tuna (mercury) and avoid salted fish...ALA, is another form of Omega 3 that the body turns into DHA but not enough to recommend in place of DHA.

The natural sources of this Omega 3 are: broccoli, dark leafy vegetables, flaxseed, spinach and walnuts. Supplementing with purified fish oil to avoid mercury toxicity is the best way to get adequate amounts of these Omega 3's. RDA is I think too low. So I take 1500mg per day.

Lastly in our supplement journey is resveratrol.

Resveratrol

Resveratrol belongs to a group of components called phytoalexins found in grapes and red wine. White wine does not have the same effect as these polyphenols are found in the skin of red grapes. Resveratrol is produced by plants to protect them against environmental stresses. Like an antibiotic, phytoalexins help protect against bacteria, fungi, harsh weather and insects. The interest in red wine was sparked by the "French Paradox"...(coined by Dr. Serge Renaud from Bordeaux University),which is the attempt to explain why the French have such a low incidence of heart disease and obesity even though they have a high fat diet and drink large amounts of red wine.

In a recent resveratrol study in the Journal of Nutritional Biochemistry, 23 adult male monkeys were divided into 3 groups.

Control Group Had A Healthy Diet

Control group "A" had a high fat and high sugar diet. And control group "B" had a high sugar and high fat diet and were also given resveratrol for two years. In year one they were given 80 mg per day and the second year they were given 480 mg per day. There was improvement in only one group and that was the last group. Although given a high fat high sugar diet this group showed marked improvements in energy metabolism, efficiency and neuro transmission, indicating improved brain signaling and more robust neurological pathways.

Dr. David Sinclair of Harvard University was able to increase the lifespan of yeast cells using resveratrol. Resveratrol activated a gene called sirtuin. This gene is a class of proteins responsible for aging, apoptosis, (the suicide of bad cells), and inflammation which compromises many bodily systems. This gene also activates the body's genetic defense mechanism. Resveratrol has the ability to turn this gene on. More importantly, resveratrol helps to assist in the repair of DNA and the regulation of genes. It directly inhibits gene expression associated with aging and age-related cardiac dysfunction. In the American Society for Microbiology, studies have indicated that resveratrol may remodel the gut by influencing the micro biota to increase the production of bile acid which decreases TMAO levels.

TMAO is trimethylamine-N-Oxide which is a risk factor for atherosclerosis. I know it is a mouthful but the bottom line is it helps the gut better than a pro-biotic does. This amazing spice is anti-cancer, anti-inflammatory, anti-diabetes, increases energy, endurance and increases protection against Alzheimer's disease. Also shown to prolong the lifespan of mice by 20%, mimics the effects of caloric restriction, lengthens longevity/anti-aging, blood sugar regulation, boosts immune system, increases muscle tone, and even helps you sleep better. Red wine, red grapes, peanut butter, dark chocolate and blueberries.

Red grapes have the most resveratrol, while blueberries have less but have other beneficial polyphenols. I supplement and take 200mg twice daily. Again, you should experiment and see what effects this supplement has and how it affects you and what benefits you may experience.

Conclusion

So yes, this is the end but actually the beginning ---- - just a starting point on your supplement journey. Thanks for taking the journey with me, hopefully it wasn't too long and I hope you found some facts interesting and helpful in your decisions regarding supplements. There are new studies daily ---- and discoveries are continually being made. The new catch phrase in vitamin delivery is called bio-availability. That is the ability of the supplement to get where it needs to go as in cell and tissue saturation.

When vitamins are given intravenously the saturation in the cell is usually 100%. Taken orally some supplements are less than 10% absorbed. So this leads us to the next break through which is manufacturing vitamins that are more readily absorbed. This is accomplished in one way by picometer technology (one trillionth of a meter) which makes extremely small molecules of the supplement thereby making it much easier to be absorbed into a cell that is very tiny itself. A good example of this is B12----this vitamin has a large molecule that the body has difficult absorbing. So the recommendation is to take a liquid form under the tongue where the tiny capillaries lay.

Besides the liquid formulas there is also the technique of chelation whereby vitamins are combined with other vitamins or minerals to aid in absorption.

This is the future of vitamins, as there are now bio-curcumin, bio-B vitamins and even liquid pico- meter magnesium which is tiny enough to be absorbed directly into the cells. This is our future of vitamin use. More and more bio-available formulas are being developed as we speak and these should be used and the efficacy determined by the individual.

My own experimentation has been that you should give a time period of at least 30 days and see how you feel. If you are improved, continue, and if not stop taking it. Every individual is different... we are not all alike. Age, sex, physical conditions all effect vitamin needs and usage. So experiment... and read as much as you can. This is your health and your body you and only you are ultimately responsible for these decisions. Don't expect to see an over worked and over scheduled physician and expect detailed assessments or recommendations.

Your body and all its functions are analogous to a symphony. All the instruments have to be tuned and the tempi have to be coordinated and the conductor must lead. Many functions in your body will work as beneficially as they can. The problem is that when we don't nurture our system the resources the body needs are lacking.... the tempo is off, the tuning of the violins, cellos and woodwinds, is off as well. The symphony will still be heard but it really won't sound as good as it should----- more like a cacophony. Your body will function but not very well. Aches, pains, arrhythmias, arthritis, diabetes, joint inflammation, headaches, nausea and general lethargy. You get the picture?

When the body has all the supplements, minerals, and nutrients it needs, then the raw material is available for the body to perform and function optimally.

This symphony of life will play brilliantly and you will benefit from a long and healthy one.

To your good health.

Robin A. Miller

Below Are A Few Of Our Highly Recommended Weight Loss Products Which Are Worth Checking Out.

The Red Tea Detox Program

http://bit.ly/2Jde8pq

The Flat Belly Fix

http://bit.ly/2TD5s0o

Printed in Great Britain
by Amazon